Epigenetics of Lifestyle

Edited By

Marcelina Párrizas

Laboratory of Diabetes and Obesity
Institut d'Investigacions Biomèdiques August Pi i Sunyer (IDIBAPS)
Barcelona, Spain

Rosa Gasa

Laboratory of Diabetes and Obesity
Institut d'Investigacions Biomèdiques August Pi i Sunyer (IDIBAPS)
Barcelona, Spain

&

Perla Kaliman

Neuroepigenetics Laboratory
Institut d'Investigacions Biomèdiques August Pi i Sunyer (IDIBAPS)
Barcelona, Spain

CONTENTS

FOREWORD

This book is a timely contribution that will be valuable to a wide range of researchers interested in the relatively new field of epigenetics. One of the difficulties of beginning, as well as pursuing, research in this field derives from its relative novelty and fast moving pace. Because the technology, concepts, and empirical research cross diverse areas and change rapidly, few have the time and ability to sustain an overview of the field. These chapters are well written, as up to date as possible, and cover a broad and important area of epigenetics in a coherent way. I think they will be especially useful to those who are entering epigenetics from other fields, or are at the start of their careers. It also has much to offer, however, for researchers who are at the cutting edge in terms of a specific question about epigenetics, but want to be more familiar with developments in the wider field.

The book focuses on the potential for epigenetics to offer mechanisms that explain the relationships between lifestyle and noncommunicable disease. This field is at the cutting edge of scientific work in the present time. We cannot know yet whether epigenetic mechanisms will turn out to be central to explanation of causal relationships and preventive interventions. Few would doubt, however, that they will at least comprise an important component.

Although the book (wisely) does not attempt to be comprehensive, it covers an array of topics and is accessible to a broad audience. It includes a well chosen selection of substantive topics within this wide area designated by the title, such that the book is useful for anyone interested in lifestyle and epigenetics, without laboriously covering every particular topic in the field. In each of the chosen areas, the authors have substantial expertise. They also do an excellent job of balancing the need to provide an introductory context in addition to presenting the most recent findings. As a result, the book is engaging, informative and remarkably readable in its entirety.

It could be useful to understand the work presented here as part of a long-term evolution, which dates back many decades but has dramatically increased its pace in recent years. The works that laid the theoretical and empirical groundwork for epidemiologic studies in this field include: in the 1960s, the theories developed by Renee Dubos, in which early development was explicitly given a central role in health and disease over the life course; in the 1970s, the work of Anders Forsdal relating infant mortality to cardiovascular mortality in later life, and the landmark study of the Dutch Hunger Winter of 1944-45 led by Zena Stein (and her husband Mervyn Susser); and in the 1980s, the work of David Barker, who built on the work of these predecessors and was pivotal in articulating the importance of such investigations for metabolic and cardiovascular disease. These, of course, only represent a small selection of the key antecedents in this field.

It is also useful for readers to keep in mind that this selection of topics falls within a broader scope of work, all of which could not be included in a single volume. With respect to nutrition, for example, nutritional supplements of folic acid have been definitively related to prevention of neural tube defects, and are now being related to prevention of other neurodevelopmental disorders (in these cases, not yet proven). Although we do not know whether the mechanism for these effects is epigenetic, it is plausible, because folic acid supplements have been widely used in animal studies of epigenetics and these studies have clearly demonstrated important epigenetic effects. In addition, early prenatal exposure to famine has been linked to schizophrenia, first in a series of studies of the Dutch Hunger Winter, and later in two separate studies based on the Chinese famine of 1959-1961. Again, epigenetic effects provide one plausible explanation for this link, and are actively being investigated.

In sum, this book provides an excellent introduction to an emerging field. I think it will be of use to readers in many disciplines. There are few similarly coherent and readable accounts that are up to date.

Ezra Susser, M.D., Ph.D.

Mailman School of Public Health
Columbia University
New York
USA

PREFACE

Recent advances in the fields of genomics and bioinformatics are evidencing the fact that genetic sequence alone can not explain how the genome regulates the development and function of complex multicellular organisms both in health and disease. The crucial role of additional layers of information piled over that of the DNA sequence has taken centre stage in the last few years and thus, decades of intensive studies on genetics have led to the emergence of epigenetics. Epigenetics comprises a number of mechanisms, such as covalent histone modifications or DNA methylation, which induce long-lasting changes in gene expression that are not encoded in the DNA sequence itself.

Epigenetics then reflects the way in which the environment in the wide sense regulates gene expression. In fact, it is becoming increasingly clear that the well-known beneficial role of a healthy lifestyle over a number of pathologies or as a pre-emptive therapy is at least in part exerted through epigenetic mechanisms. Likewise, changes in chromatin structure may lie beneath some of the altered behavioral patterns usually associated with depression and addiction.

The current research on epigenetics is thus providing us with a fresh outlook to interpret genetic information. Fascinating new data suggest that we are a product of our genes but we can also influence them through our choices and experiences. When designing this book, our main intention has been to provide a comprehensive view of how lifestyle affects chromatin and, as a result, gene function and ultimately organismal fitness. The chapters of this book have been written by eminent scientists actively working in the fields they review. Following an introductory chapter in which the main concepts and background regarding epigenetics are discussed, there are chapters devoted to describe the epigenetic impact of nutrition, stress, addiction, exposure to chemicals and pollutants and how some of these epigenetic marks regulate brain functions such as learning and memory. In summary, our intention is to approach epigenetics from a fresh perspective and present the reader with the latest and most significant research in the field of epigenetics and lifestyle.

Marcelina Párrizas
Rosa Gasa
Perla Kaliman
Institut d'Investigacions Biomèdiques August Pi i Sunyer (IDIBAPS)
Barcelona
Spain

List of Contributors

Jorge A. Alegría-Torres, Ph.D.
Departamento de Toxicología Ambiental
Facultad de Medicina
Universidad Autónoma de San Luis Potosí
San Luis Potosí, México

Andrea Baccarelli M.D., Ph.D.
Exposure, Epidemiology and Risk Program
Department of Environmental Health
Harvard School of Public Health
Boston, Massachusetts, USA

Valentina Bollati, Ph.D.
Center of Molecular and Genetic Epidemiology
Department of Environmental and Occupational Health
Università degli Studi di Milano
Fondazione IRCCS Ospedale Maggiore Policlinico, Mangiagalli e Regina Elena
Milan, Italy

Graham C. Burdge, Ph.D.
Human Development and Health
Faculty of Medicine
University of Southampton
Southampton, United Kingdom

Andrew Collins, B.Sc.
Henry Wellcome Laboratories for Integrative Neuroscience and Endocrinology
University of Bristol
Bristol, United Kingdom

Rosa Gasa, Ph.D.
Laboratory of Diabetes and Obesity
Institut d'Investigacions Biomèdiques August Pi i Sunyer (IDIBAPS)
Barcelona, Spain

María Gutièrrez-Mecinas, Ph.D.
Henry Wellcome Laboratories for Integrative Neuroscience and Endocrinology

University of Bristol
Bristol, United Kingdom

Perla Kaliman, Ph.D.
Neuroepigenetics Laboratory
Institut d'Investigacions Biomèdiques August Pi i Sunyer (IDIBAPS)
Barcelona, Spain

Karen A. Lillycrop, Ph.D.
School of Biological Sciences
Faculty of Natural and Environmental Sciences
University of Southampton
Southampton, United Kingdom

Isabelle M. Mansuy, Ph.D.
Brain Research Institute
University of Zürich and Swiss Federal Institute of Technology
Zürich/Switzerland

Marta Miquel, Ph.D.
Psychobiology Unit
Universitat Jaume I
Castellón de la Plana, Spain

Marcelina Párrizas, Ph.D.
Laboratory of Diabetes and Obesity
Institut d'Investigacions Biomèdiques August Pi i Sunyer (IDIBAPS)
Barcelona, Spain

Johannes M.H.M. Reul, Ph.D.
Henry Wellcome Laboratories for Integrative Neuroscience and Endocrinology
University of Bristol
Bristol, United Kingdom

Bechara J. Saab, Ph.D.
Brain Research Institute
University of Zürich and Swiss Federal Institute of Technology
Zürich/Switzerland

Carla Sanchis-Segura, Ph.D.
Psychobiology Unit
Universitat Jaume I
Castellón de la Plana, Spain

Ezra Susser, M.D. Dr. P.H.
Mailman School of Public Health,
Columbia University, New York,
NY 10032-3727, USA.

Alexandra F. Trollope, Ph.D.
Henry Wellcome Laboratories for Integrative Neuroscience and Endocrinology
University of Bristol
Bristol, United Kingdom

2

CHAPTER 1

Epigenetics of Lifestyle: The Plasticity of the Genetic Information

Marcelina Párrizas[1,2,*], Rosa Gasa[1,2,*] and Perla Kaliman[3,*]

[1]Laboratory of Diabetes and Obesity, Institut d'Investigacions Biomèdiques August Pi i Sunyer (IDIBAPS), Hospital Clínic, University of Barcelona; [2] CIBER de diabetes y enfermedades metabólicas asociadas (CIBERDEM) and [3]Systems Neuroscience, Psychoneuroepigenetics Laboratory, IDIBAPS, Hospital Clínic, University of Barcelona, Barcelona, Spain

Abstract: The concept of epigenetics refers nowadays to the long-lasting and inheritable gene expression states that are established in the absence of a change in the DNA sequence itself. The fast progress of the field in later times has provided scientists with novel understanding on how the environment in the wide sense, including nutrition, exercise, even behavior of the organisms, participates in the regulation of gene expression. The molecular mechanisms that mediate epigenetic regulation are principally DNA methylation, the post-translational modifications of the histones and the regulation by non-coding RNAs. They are intimately related to cell differentiation and developmental plasticity and relay environmental influences to the cell nucleus, thus bridging the gap between lifestyle and the genome. In this introductory chapter we offer a general vision of the well-documented effects of lifestyle choices and environmental impact on gene expression and present the reader with a general overview of the better known epigenetic mechanisms and the techniques most often used to study them.

Keywords: Chromatin, DNA methylation, histones, lifestyle.

1.1. LIFESTYLE AND HEALTH

A pillar of the ancient wisdom of health and healing was the understanding that experience and life choices shape the human body and mind. Greeks in the sixth to fourth centuries BC developed a medical and philosophical school of thought that stated that health and disease were influenced by behavior and environment. Indeed, Western and Eastern sages such as Hippocrates of Kos (Greek physician,

*****Address correspondence to Marcelina Párrizas:** Laboratori de Diabetes i Obesitat, CEK, Roselló 149-153, Barcelona 08036, Spain; Email: badcell@gmail.com; **Rosa Gasa:** Laboratori de Diabetes i Obesitat, CEK, Roselló 149-153, Barcelona 08036, Spain; Tel: +34932275400, ext 4552/4313; Fax: +34933129409; Email: rgasa@clinic.ub.es and **Perla Kaliman:** Psychoneuroepigenetics Laboratory, Córcega 176, Barcelona 08036, Spain; Email: pkaliman@clinic.ub.es

4th century BC) and Patanjali (Indian philosopher, 2nd century BC) emphasized that maintenance of good health was intimately linked to social and physical environment, diet, living habits and even thinking patterns [1, 2].

Thousands of years later, modern science has begun to corroborate some of these ancient concepts by using sophisticated technologies. In the last few decades, it has become evident that numerous age-related pathologies, including cardiovascular disease, type 2 diabetes and neurodegenerative disorders such as Alzheimer's disease, are either caused or aggravated by lifestyle factors through strong interactions with the genetic information. It is noteworthy that such pathologies are among the ten leading causes of mortality in Western societies. Fortunately, the counterpart also seems to be true: with increasing frequency, scientists are finding that for some of these diseases, lifestyle modifications can be preventive or even improve the outcomes of classical pharmacological therapies, thus helping reduce medical treatment in many cases [3-6]. In this context, there is a growing trend of scientific research devoted to understanding the physiological and cellular responses induced by lifestyle, with the ultimate objective of identifying new therapeutic targets and developing multimodal health-care strategies that meet the needs of an aging population.

It is now accepted that gene expression is modulated by the interaction of "nature" and "nurture". What scientists mean by "nature" is the influence of the information coded in the inherited genome, which differs between subjects mainly due to slight variations in the DNA sequence (polymorphisms). These variations may cause changes in protein expression and function, leading to direct effects on the phenotype (the physical, physiological, and behavioral characteristics of the individual) and influencing its susceptibility to the environment. "Nurture" refers to the impact of personal experiences (including environmental exposures since the moment of conception and lifestyle) on health.

1.2. LIFESTYLE INFLUENCES GENE EXPRESSION

It is widely documented that a sedentary and stressful lifestyle accompanied by a pro-inflammatory and pro-oxidant diet (*i.e.* based on animal-derived products, highly processed foods and those rich in saturated fatty acids) forms the basis of most chronic diseases associated with aging that affect a high proportion of the population. For this reason, over the last few years, the scientific community has been investing increasing efforts and resources in the study of how particular lifestyle conditions modify gene expression patterns with the ultimate purpose of providing new tools for disease prevention and treatment. For instance, the impact of mild physical exercise on gene expression and its correlation with neurophysiological variables has been confirmed in humans and in animal models by using microarray technology that allows simultaneous analysis of thousands of genes. Indeed, animals voluntarily trained in a running wheel showed important changes in cellular, cardiometabolic and neurochemical parameters. In adult animals, physical training has been shown to: (i) enhance performance in learning and memory tasks [7-9]; (ii) enhance survival [10]; (iii) increase neuronal proliferation [11-13]; (iv) affect neuronal structure and the functionality of cellular mechanisms associated with learning processes [14, 15]; and (v) reduce cardiometabolic risk [16]. In mice, brain gene expression is sensitive to physical exercise, particularly in the hippocampus, which plays a key role in learning and memory processes. These findings are particularly relevant because the hippocampus is especially susceptible to dysfunctional and degenerative processes during aging or in Alzheimer's disease, and it is involved in the regulation of mood and antidepressant responses [17-19].

Nutrition also influences gene expression patterns and there is a novel and promising field in biomedical research known as "Nutrigenomics," which applies state-of-the-art molecular genetics technologies to nutritional studies. Plant-derived molecules such as curcumin (one of the main ingredients of Indian curry), resveratrol (present in black grape seeds and red wine), and catechins (abundant compounds of green tea) have emerged from human epidemiological studies as efficient molecules for the prevention of Alzheimer's disease, and this has been confirmed in cellular and animal models [20]. Among them, resveratrol also has the potential to reduce the risk of cardiometabolic diseases and to prolong life expectancy in a wide spectrum of organisms ranging from yeast and fruit flies to mammals, through a mechanism involving changes in the activity of a group of conserved enzymes known as the sirtuins. Sirtuins bind to and modify a number of key transcription factors (such as the PPARs, PGC-1α and members of the

FoxO family) that regulate metabolism through specific changes in gene expression [21]. Synthetic curcumin analogues have recently been shown to inhibit prostate cancer proliferation by enhancing the degradation of the androgen receptor, which modulates the transcription of target genes involved in the progression of the disease [22]. Similarly, green tea may exert a positive effect on vascular function through its polyphenols, especially epigallocatechin-3-gallate. It has been suggested that these effects are mediated by changes in transcription of phase II detoxifying and antioxidant defense enzymes in vascular cells [23].

Stress reactivity during life also has a powerful impact on the way our genes are expressed, and in the long term stress can influence our physical and mental health. Indeed, living in chronically stressful conditions has a negative influence on many cellular responses. A history of poor maternal care in early life, childhood abuse, stressful life events and adverse socioeconomic environments can influence the structure and function of the brain through neuroplastic mechanisms which involve changes in specific gene expression patterns, as a consequence of which emotional, cognitive and cell aging processes may be affected. For instance, chronic stress raises extracellular levels of glutamate in the hippocampus of rats [24], and alters the expression of glutamate receptor subunits [25] and the levels of glial glutamate transporter 1 [26], all of which are associated with mood disorders [27]. The counterpart of the stress response has been defined as the "relaxation response" and its elicitation, which can be trained through practices such as mindfulness-based mental training, is associated with physiological and gene expression changes [28]. Indeed, mind-body techniques such as yoga and meditation were already used to prevent and treat diseases in ancient cultures but it was not until recently that they have been shown to be relevant therapeutic tools [29]. Interestingly, a recent study has revealed that subjects that received a training of 8 weeks which included 20 minutes per day of relaxation response practice, showed specific gene expression changes in cellular pathways involved in metabolic regulation and oxidative stress [30].

Environmental pollutants as well as substance abuse also modulate gene responses. These pollutants are introduced to the atmosphere by humans or by nature itself, for instance due to the eruption of volcanoes or forest fires. These substances can affect the composition of soil, water or air. Air pollution, caused by the accumulation of substances such as nitrogen oxides, ozone, carbon monoxide or fine particulate matter, has been associated with increased incidence of asthma, chronic obstructive pulmonary disease, cardiopulmonary diseases, lung cancer and mortality [31]. To mention just one example, ozone pollution (a byproduct of atmospheric reactions but also of electronic devices such as copy machines and laser printers) can induce a cascade of oxidation, inflammation and cell injury through activation of transcription factors such as NF-κB [32] and c-jun [33]. While air pollution is difficult to control for those of us living in large cities and dependent on technology, exposure to harmful substances can be considered in many cases as life choices, for example the consumption of tobacco, alcohol and drugs. In that respect, it is now recognized that repeated consumption of addictive substances can generate brain neuroadaptive reward networks through the induction of specific transcription factors (*i.e.* Fos family) that promote dependence, craving and relapse after withdrawal [34].

As a whole, the studies mentioned above indicate that lifestyle habits and environmental exposures exert physiological and cognitive effects which are mediated by changes in transcriptional profiles, although in most cases the molecular mechanisms responsible are still unknown. During the last few decades, scientists have started to show that both lifestyle and environment have an impact on health and disease at least in part through the addition of new layers of information on top of our inherited genetic code. The discovery of these mechanisms, which are referred to as *epigenetic,* has given rise to a new biomedical and social paradigm based on the concept of the plasticity of genetic information.

1.3. EPIGENETICS: DEFINITION AND CONCEPTS

The deciphering of the structure of DNA by Watson and Crick in 1953 [35, 36] and the subsequent breaking of the genetic code by Marshall Niremberg and colleagues in 1961 [37] brought with them the beginning of the genomic era and the exaltation of DNA as the "blueprint" for life. The pace of discovery accelerated from that moment onwards, peaking with the conclusion of the first draft of the human genome sequence in June 2000, which gave the scientists access to a wealth of information that is still being thoroughly mined today [38,

39]. In the intervening years, the genome sequences of several model organisms as well as others with economical and biomedical interests have been completed, providing us with insights on the mechanisms of normal and pathological cell development. Recently, the first artificial genome has been built. Scientists at the J. Craig Venter Institute in Rockville (Maryland, USA) synthesized the complete genome of the bacteria *Mycoplasma mycoides* and transplanted it into an *M.capricolum* recipient cell, which then acquired phenotypic characteristics of *M.mycoides* and was able to grow and self-replicate [40]. This technical prowess goes a long way to show that the primary sequence of DNA contains the necessary information to direct the development and function of a living being. At least this seems to be true for unicellular organisms, although the fact is that the synthetic DNA was inserted into a cell already containing a full complement of proteins and other components that also participate in cellular function.

However, the situation is much more complex in the case of multicellular organisms. Access to the complete primary sequence of the human genome has highlighted the fact that genetic sequence alone cannot explain how the genome regulates the development and function of a wide assortment of cell types with highly specialized functions and wildly different phenotypes, all of them arising from the same precursor cell and containing the same basic DNA sequence. The DNA of eukaryotic cells is over 300 times longer than that of bacteria. This means that, if extended, the human genome would measure close to 2 m in length. This long molecule must be encapsulated in a cell nucleus a few micrometers in diameter, thus requiring a considerable degree of compaction. To achieve this, DNA is associated with proteins, of which the histones represent the main fraction, constituting the chromatin (Fig. **1**). The main implication of the highly compacted status of DNA in eukaryotic cells is that, contrarily to what happens in prokaryotic cells, access of transcription factors and other regulatory proteins to DNA is not granted by default, but controlled by the structure and degree of compaction of chromatin at any given region. Thus, in eukaryotic cells, both DNA itself and its associated proteins are targeted by an array of molecular modifications that influence gene expression without altering the primary sequence of DNA by either favoring or denying access of regulatory proteins to DNA [41]. These additional layers of information piled over that of DNA are what constitute the field of study of epigenetics.

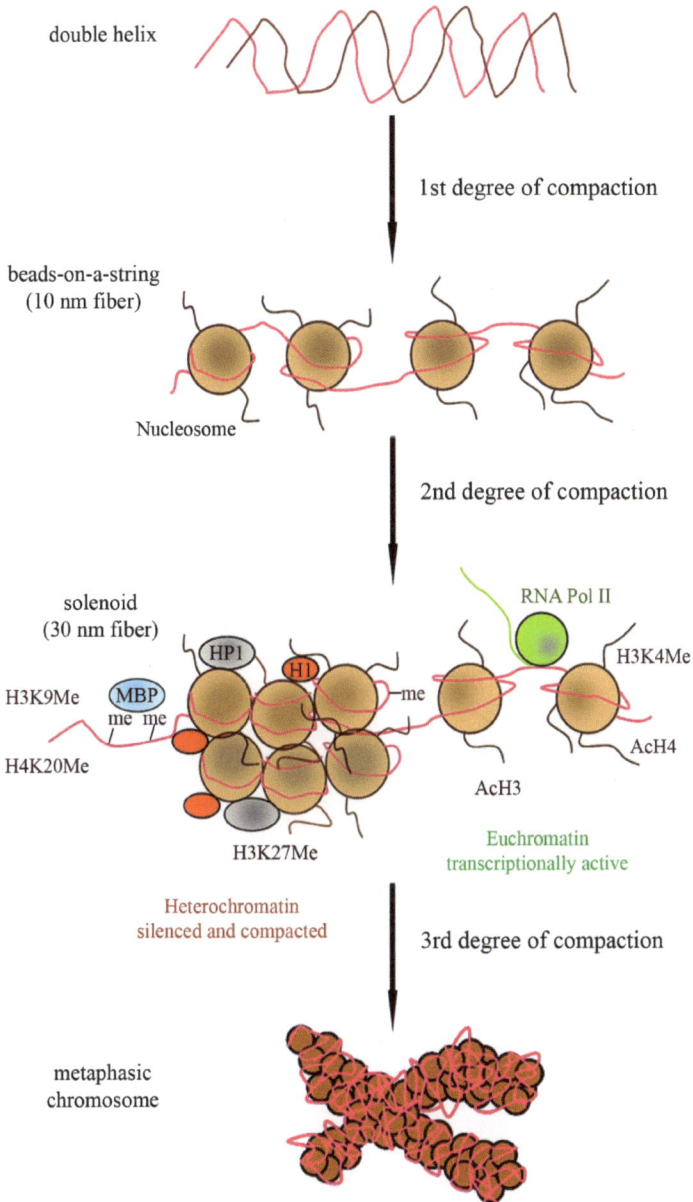

Figure 1: The double helix of DNA carries the genetic information. In eukaryotic cells, DNA is associated with structural proteins, among them the histones, constituting the chromatin. The main unit of the chromatin is the nucleosome, which consists of 147 bp of DNA wrapped around a core of eight histone proteins (2 units each of histones H2A, H2B, H3 and H4). Nucleosomes distributed along the DNA chain represent a first degree of compaction, giving rise to a chromatin fiber of 10 nm in diameter that is usually known as the "*beads-on-a-string*" structure. A second degree of compaction is obtained when other proteins are bound to this basic structure, such as

histone H1, which binds to the DNA regions in between nucleosomes (the "linker" DNA). A fiber of 30 nm in diameter, the solenoid, is then constituted. The maximal degree of compaction is found in the condensed chromosomes during mitosis, when all DNA-related processes (transcription, DNA repair) must be stopped. Chromatin controls access to the information stored in the DNA and, accordingly, two types of chromatin can be distinguished: *heterochromatin* is heavily compacted and mostly inactive, whereas *euchromatin* displays a more open, transcriptionally active, structure. Epigenetic marks differentiate heterochromatin from euchromatin. Thus, in heterochromatin, histones are hypoacetylated and enriched in methylation marks associated with gene silencing (methylation of H3K9, H3K27 and H4K20), as well as high levels of DNA methylation, which usually results in transcriptional silencing. Repressive histone marks and methylated DNA recruit proteins that help obstruct access to DNA, such as heterochromatin protein 1 (HP1) that recognizes and binds to methylated H3K9 or the methyl CpG binding proteins such as MeCP2 or MBD2 that associate with methylated DNA. Euchromatin, on the other hand, is enriched in histone acetylation and methylation marks that correlate with transcription such as methylation of H3K4. Moreover, nucleosomes are less compacted than in hetrochromatin and access of transcription factors and the basal transcriptional machinery (RNA Polymerase II and associated factors) to the DNA is allowed, thus favoring active transcription.

The concept of epigenetics currently refers to the cellular mechanisms that control somatically, and sometimes transgenerationally, inheritable gene expression states that are established in the absence of a change in the DNA sequence itself [42, 43]. However, for the purposes of this book, we will follow the definition recently provided by the Epigenomics Program of the National Institutes of Health (NIH) (http://nihroadmap.nih.gov/epigenomics/index.asp) that defined epigenetics as referring to "both heritable changes in gene activity and expression (in the progeny of cells or of individuals) and also stable, long-term alterations in the transcriptional potential of a cell that are not necessarily heritable". We thus acknowledge as epigenetic those long-lasting changes in gene expression that are not inherited. Interestingly, one of the defining features of epigenetic mechanisms is that they are theoretically reversible, contrarily to the primary sequence of DNA, which is unchanged throughout lifetime except for occasional mutations.

Epigenetic processes play a crucial role in the establishment and maintenance of cell identity by selectively activating or repressing transcription of subsets of tissue-specific genes. For this reason, epigenetics is a crucial element in the regulation of cell differentiation and transformation, but also in the response to environmental signals. The molecular mechanisms that mediate epigenetic regulation are principally DNA methylation, chromatin remodeling, the post-translational modifications of the histones, the replacement of histones by histone variants, the control of the higher-level organization of chromatin within the nucleus and the regulation by non-coding RNAs (reviewed in reference [41]). Of these, DNA methylation and the covalent modification of histones are the best studied to date. These two processes influence each other and together regulate the establishment and maintenance of epigenetic events capable of modulating the fate of the cell and its response to environmental signals [44, 45].

1.3.1. DNA Methylation

The structure of DNA is covalently modified by base methylation in virtually all cells and organisms. This process is crucial for normal organismal development and cellular differentiation as it regulates vital cellular processes such as transcription, X chromosome inactivation and genomic imprinting. In fact, DNA methylation is among the most stable epigenetic marks, ensuring tissue-specific gene expression in a heritable manner throughout embryogenesis. Hence, it is not surprising that aberrant DNA methylation associates with the etiology of human disease, in particular with developmental disorders and cancer. Furthermore, especially relevant to the topic of this book, an increasing amount of data generated during this last decade illustrates how DNA methylation patterns may be modified in response to specific environmental conditions, thus making this modification an important contributor to the epigenetics of lifestyle.

In humans, methylation of cytosine DNA residues is the most widely studied epigenetic modification. It involves the addition of a methyl group to the position 5 of the cytosine pyrimidine ring. This occurs almost exclusively within cytosine-guanine dinucleotides (CpG) in somatic cells [46] whereas it is also found in non-CpG sequences in embryonic stem cells [47]. Remarkably, the distribution of CpGs throughout the genome is not homogeneous. Rather, CpGs are overrepresented in repetitive sequences in transposons and pericentromeric satellite regions and in endogenous retroviral DNA. In these regions, DNA methylation is thought to prevent their activation and mobility and, consequently, guarantee genomic stability. In agreement, cancerous cells are largely depleted of CpG methylation at repetitive sequences and intronic regions, and this phenomenon has been correlated with reactivation of transposons and loss of imprinted genes, all of which contribute to development of cancer [48].

On the contrary, in the rest of the mammalian genome CpGs are often underrepresented. This is most likely due to the spontaneous deamination of methylated cytosine to thymidine that has resulted in the progressive substitution of CpG for TpG dinucleotides during evolution. A notorious exception are the 5'-ends of nearly half of human genes where CpGs concentrate in short stretches or clusters (500–2000 bp) known as CpG islands [49]. Most CpG islands are found unmethylated in both transcriptionally active and silent genes, which indicates that DNA methylation may be dispensable for general gene repression *in vivo* [50]. Nonetheless, absence of methylation in the CpG islands within the promoter region of a gene seems to be a prerequisite for its transcriptional activation. Importantly, within a subgroup of promoters associated with tissue-specific and germ-line genes, CpG islands are methylated as part of normal development and, when this happens, these genes are stably repressed. Conversely, in cancerous cells, selective hypermethylation at the CpG-rich promoters of key tumor supressor genes and critical regulatory miRNAs is observed. This phenomenon associates with silencing of these genes and constitutes a crucial step towards tumor formation [48]. Lastly, DNA hypermethylation is also linked to gene silencing in genomic imprinting and X-chromosome inactivation in females.

1.3.1.1. The DNA Methylation Pathway

DNA methylation is carried out by a group of evolutionarily conserved enzymes called DNA methyltransferases (DNMTs). These enzymes can be classified into two major types: *de novo* and maintenance methyltransferases. The first group, which includes DNMT3A and DNMT3B, establishes the DNA methylation patterns during embryonic development whereas the second group, epitomized by DNMT1, copies these patterns to the complementary strand of hemimethylated DNA generated from DNA replication during subsequent cell divisions. Mouse models deficient for all three genes have been generated and display embryonic or early postnatal lethality, thus supporting the fundamental role of this epigenetic modification in development [51, 52]. Two more DNMTs, DNMT2 and DNMT3L, have been identified in mammals. DNMT2 is the most widely conserved DNMT but, paradoxically, it is also the less understood. Indeed, available data are contradictory with regard to its roles as a DNA or RNA methyltransferase [53]. Furthermore, *Dnmt2* knockout mice are viable and display no obvious major phenotypes [54]. On the other hand, DNMT3L, which is homologous to DNMT3A/B but lacks a functional catalytic domain, is believed to indirectly affect DNA methylation by recruiting DNMT3A to specific DNA sites [55]. *Dnmt3L*-deficient mice are born infertile and display severe germ cells anomalies [56].

The methyl groups added to DNA by the action of the DNMTs protrude into the major groove of DNA, providing novel functional moieties available for molecular interactions. A highly conserved family of DNA-binding proteins which share a common motif, the methyl CpG binding domain (MBD), specifically recognizes and binds methyl-cytosine [57, 58]. These proteins are thought to be pivotal for "reading" DNA methylation patterns and convert them into appropriate functional states. Hence, they are critical components of DNA methylation-dependent gene repression. Gene silencing by MBD family members is accomplished by at least two different mechanisms. First, MBDs may interfere with transcription by preventing the binding of transcription factors to their cognate DNA sequences. On the other hand, possibly concomitantly, MBDs may contribute to the reorganization of chromatin into a transcriptionally repressed state through recruitment of histone modifying enzymes such as histone deacetylases or methyltransferases [59].

Despite the reported stability of DNA methylation, regulated reprogramming of this modification is observed during development, in particular at gametogenesis and after fertilization when extensive demethylation and remethylation events take place [60]. In addition, localized DNA demethylation has been observed later at specific genes, mostly when and where differentiation requires their activation [61, 62]. In both scenarios, loss of methylation appears to entail two distinct mechanisms that most likely work together: a passive mechanism resulting from the absence of maintenance methylation after replication and an active mechanism involving removal of methylcytosines [55]. Although the existence of mammalian enzymes that can directly remove this modified nucleotide has been controversial, current models propose that DNA demethylation in mammals is mediated at least in part by a base excision repair pathway where the AID/APOBEC family of deaminases converts 5-methylcytosine to thymine followed by G/T mismatch repair by the DNA glycosylase TDG and MBD4 [63].

1.3.1.2. Techniques to Study DNA Methylation

The recognition of the fundamental role of DNA methylation in human health and disease has impelled the development of a wide range of methodologies designed to provide quantitative and qualitative information on DNA methylation profiles. While the first studies concentrated on the measurement of the overall level of methylcytosines in the genome using chromatographic methods and methyl accepting capacity assays [64], later efforts have been largely directed towards the characterization of gene-specific DNA methylation states. Two different approaches have been instrumental to achieve this goal: (i) the use of methylation-sensitive restriction enzymes that digest only unmethylated DNA and (ii) bisulfite modification of DNA which converts unmethylated C to T but leaves methylated C residues unaffected. In either case, specific genes can then be studied by end-point or real time PCR employing primers designed to amplify the genes of interest. For bisulfite-treated DNA, primer pairs are designed to be 'methylated-specific' by targeting sequences complementing only unconverted 5-methylcytosines, or 'unmethylated-specific' by complementing thymines converted from unmethylated cytosines (termed MSP methodology). In addition to candidate gene approaches, both methods can be used in combination with whole genome strategies in order to generate comprehensive unbiased maps of DNA methylation profiles across a variety of biological settings. For example, fragments resulting from the digestion with methylation-sensitive restriction enzymes can be hybridized to high density genomic microarrays, whereas bisulfite-modified DNA may serve as input material for high-throughput sequencing (HTS) techniques (Fig. **2**).

An important drawback inherent to the restriction-based methods is that only particular sequence motifs can be analyzed because specific restriction sites are required to be present. Also, inefficient bisulfite treatment may result in incomplete C to T conversion and compromised data. In an attempt to overcome these limitations, alternative methods have been designed that rely on the selective interaction of certain proteins with methylated DNA [65]. In this regard, the specific binding of MBD proteins to methylcytosines has been exploited in a variety of strategies such as MBD-bound affinity columns and chromatin immunoprecipitation (ChIP) techniques using antibodies raised against members of this protein family [66] (for more detailed explanation on ChIP see section

1.3.2.1). More recently, a new technology termed MeDip has been established that uses an antibody against 5-methylcytosine to directly immunoprecipitate methylated DNA [67]. The precipitated DNA is then used for individual analysis of the methylation status of a particular gene by PCR or for global methylation analysis using microarrays or HTS as stated previously.

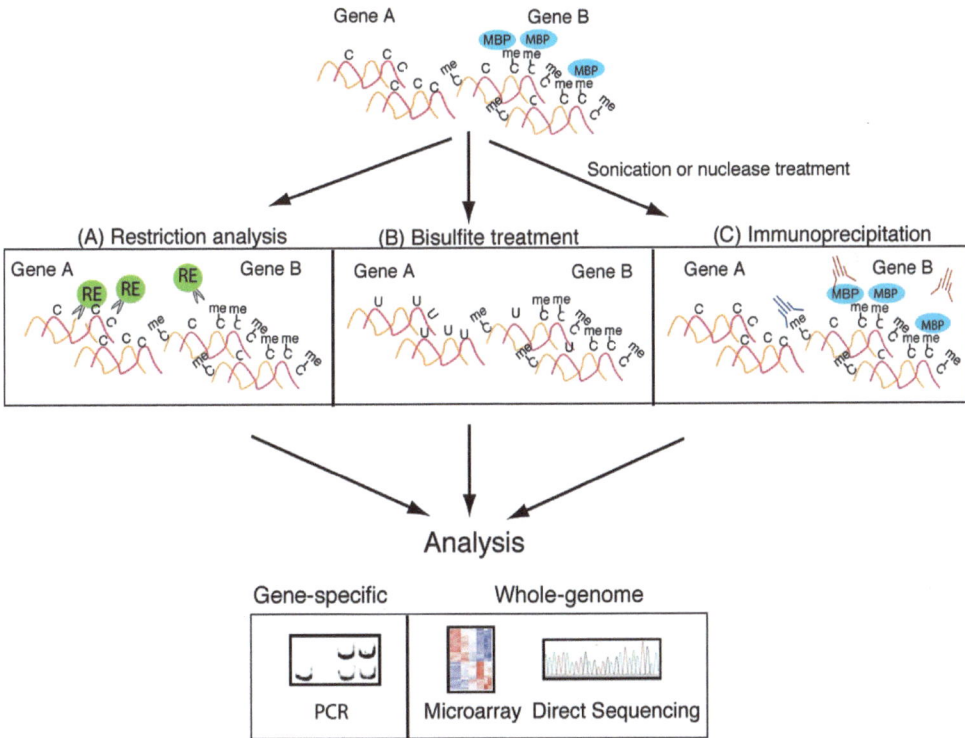

Figure 2: Outline of the three main methodologies used to study gene-specific DNA methylation. In (A), a methylation-sensitive restriction enzyme (RE) is used to digest un-methylated DNA. In (B), treatment of DNA with sodium bisulfite converts un-methylated cytosines to uracils while leaving methylated cytosines unaltered. In (C), antibodies recognizing either methyl-cytosine (depicted in blue) or methyl-cytosine binding proteins/MBPs (depicted in red) are used to immunoprecipate DNA. In all three methods, the obtained DNA can be analysed by traditional PCR amplification with selected primers for specific genes. Additionally, in order to identify unknown methylation hot-spots or methylated CpG islands in the genome, the obtained DNA can be used as input DNA for genome-wide screen methods such as DNA microarrays or direct sequencing.

1.3.2. Post-Translational Modifications of the Histones

Methylation is the only epigenetic mark that affects the DNA molecule itself. In contrast, a broad collection of epigenetic modifications targets the histone proteins, which together with DNA, make up chromatin. As mentioned earlier, DNA is highly compacted in eukaryotic cells. The first degree of compaction of DNA is the folding of a stretch 147 bp long over a core of eight histone proteins, constituting a nucleosome (Fig. **1**). Nucleosomes are the basic units of chromatin and consist of two molecules each of histones H2A, H2B, H3 and H4. Histones are small basic proteins with a C-terminal histone fold domain that regulates histone-histone and histone-DNA interactions, and an N-terminal unstructured tail that protrudes out of the nucleosome and contains a high percentage of lysine and arginine residues. This tail is the main target of a number of transcriptional co-regulators that have the capacity to enzymatically modify histones by acetylation, methylation, phosphorylation, sumoylation, deimination or ubiquitylation [68, 69] (Fig. **3**). Adding a layer of complexity, a number of histone-modifying enzymes also target non-histone proteins, such as sequence-specific transcription factors or members of the basal transcriptional machinery, thus broadening their range of influence upon gene activity [68].

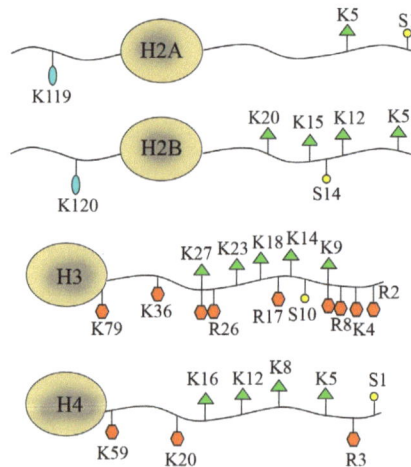

Figure 3: Schematic representation of some of the best studied enzymatic modifications of the four core histones. Acetylation (green triangles) is usually associated with gene activity, whereas the result of lysine or arginine methylation (red hexagons), serine or threonine phosphorylation (yellow circles) and lysine ubiquitination (blue ellipses) depends on the modified residue. Possible outcomes include not only transcriptional activation or silencing, but also DNA repair (H3K14 acetylation, H4K5 acetylation), apoptosis (H2BS14 phosphorylation), histone deposition during DNA replication (H4K12 acetylation) or chromosome condensation during mitosis (H3S10 phosphorylation, H2AS1 phosphorylation). K: lysine; R: arginine; S: serine; T: threonine.

Numerous reports have shown a clear link between the pattern of histone modifications in the chromatin of a given gene and its transcriptional status. Thus, histone lysine acetylation is usually related to gene activation [70, 71], whereas arginine and lysine methylation result in different outcomes, depending on the modified residue [69]. Hence, global analyses of histone lysine methylation have shown that methylation of lysine 4 of histone 3 (H3K4) usually correlates with gene activation [72-74], whereas methylation of H3K9 or H3K27 associates with transcriptional silencing [75, 76]. Moreover, lysine residues can be mono-, di- or trimethylated *in vivo*, thus providing a further layer of complexity and exponentially increasing functional diversity [75].

The observed correlation between specific histone modifications and particular DNA-dependent processes, including gene expression, and the fact that the presence or absence of particular modifications often affects the presence or absence of other modifications led to the statement of the histone code hypothesis [77], which postulates that the pattern of histone post-translational modifications in a locus considerably extends the amount of information conveyed by the genomic code, by modulating access to the DNA or actively recruiting transcriptional regulators. The existence of a wide variety of protein domains that specifically recognize modified histones supports this hypothesis. Thus, chromodomains, PHD fingers and TUDOR domains recognize methylated lysine residues; bromodomains bind to acetylated lysines, and 14-3-3 domains recognize phosphorylated serines [69]. Moreover, residue discrimination is highly sensitive. For instance, the chromodomain of heterochromatin protein 1 (HP1) specifically recognizes and binds to methylated H3K9 [75], thus resulting in gene silencing and heterochromatin formation and spreading, as HP1 interacts with the H3K9 methyltransferase SUV39H1 thus bringing H3K9 methyltransferase activity to a region already enriched in this modified residue. The double bromodomain of TBP-associated factor TAF1, on the other hand, recognizes histone H3 acetylated a both K9 and K14, thus providing a mechanistic explanation linking histone acetylation and transcription [78].

Histone acetylation is highly dynamic [79, 80], being its global levels a result of the balance of the activities of opposing enzymes histone acetyltransferases (HATs) and histone deacetylases (HDACs). Histone lysine methylation, on the other hand, was until recently considered to be a permanent mark as no demethylases had been identified [81]. However, the recent discovery of two classes of histone lysine demethylases [82-86] established the dynamic nature of this modification. The first histone demethylase described, lysine-specific histone demethylase 1 (LSD1), is an amine oxidase that mediates histone demethylation *via* a FAD-dependent oxidative reaction and has been found to be associated with a number of corepressor complexes [87, 88]. In agreement with these data, LSD1 has been shown to specifically demethylate *in vitro* mono- and dimethylated H3K4, and has been suggested to mediate gene repression *in vivo* by maintaining an unmethylated H3K4 status on a set of target promoters [83, 87]. Other studies have shown that, depending on its associated partners, LSD1 can also act as a co-activator by demethylating mono- and dimethylated H3K9 [89, 90]. However, by the nature of its demethylase reaction, LSD1 is unable to demethylate trimethylated lysine residues. Thus enter the *jumonji* family of demethylases [82]. These histone demethylases remove methyl groups from lysines by means of a hydroxylation reaction that can target trimethylated as well as di- and monomethylated lysine residues [91].

Intriguingly, functional interplay between histone and DNA methylation has been described. In *Neurospora crassa,* histone H3K9 methylation is required for DNA methylation and replacement of the residue by a leucine or an arginine results in loss of DNA methylation [92]. In mammals, the histone demethylase LSD1 demethylates and thus stabilizes DNA methyltransferase DNMT1, so that in absence of LSD1, DNMT1 decreases and DNA methylation is eventually lost [93]. Histone methyltransferase G9a, on the other hand, recruits DNMT3a and DNMT3b to DNA, thus regulating DNA methylation independently of its histone methyltransferase activity [94]. Hence, two different silencing epigenetic modifications team up to ensure proper gene repression.

1.3.2.1. Methods Used to Study the Post-Translational Modifications of the Histones

Classical *in vitro* methodologies such as electrophoretic mobility shift assays (EMSA) that detect binding of transcriptional regulators to naked DNA are still useful in many situations but result insufficient to study the role of chromatin as a major regulatory element in transcription. Thus, in the last few years, the chromatin immunoprecipitation (ChIP) assay has been established as a powerful method to examine the access of nuclear proteins to their target promoters in the natural chromatin environment, as well as to study the covalent modifications of the histones that constitute the nucleosomes spanning genomic regions of interest (Fig. **4**) [95]. The ChIP procedure is based on the ability of formaldehyde to reversibly crosslink amino and imino groups of both amino acids and DNA that are found within a maximal distance of 2 Å from each other [96]. This short range of action warrants that the crosslinks generated in this way represent direct interactions taking place in the cell at a determined time-point [80]. By using a specific antibody directed against a particular transcription factor or a modified histone it is possible to precipitate the protein of interest, pulling along with it the DNA sequences to which this protein is bound. In order to achieve this, the DNA should have been previously fragmented randomly into small pieces ensuring that the co-precipitated DNA actually represents the sequences found in the close vicinity of the selected protein. The co-precipitated DNA can be analyzed by different techniques. The straightest analysis is to perform semi-quantitative endpoint or real-time PCR using primers designed to detect the presence or absence of a region of interest in the precipitate. In recent times, global analysis of histone modifications or transcription factor binding has been performed by coupling ChIP with microarray hybridization of direct sequencing of the precipitated DNA [97, 98]. These strategies allow a nonbiased analysis of the sample, thus obtaining global profiles of histone modifications or transcription factor binding and identifying genes of interest that would not have been found otherwise.

1.3.3. Non-Coding RNAs

Genome-wide analyses of transcription in humans and other complex organisms have uncovered the existence of a large plethora of RNA molecules that are not translated into proteins, commonly referred to as non-coding RNAs (ncRNAs) [99, 100]. In fact, in the human transcriptome, protein-coding transcripts barely account for 25% of the DNA that is being transcribed [101]. In this same line, it is estimated that more than 90% of each base position in the genome is transcribed on at least one strand [102]. Apart from the long-known transfer RNA (tRNA), ribosomal RNA (rRNA), spliceosomal RNAs (snRNAs/uRNAs) and small

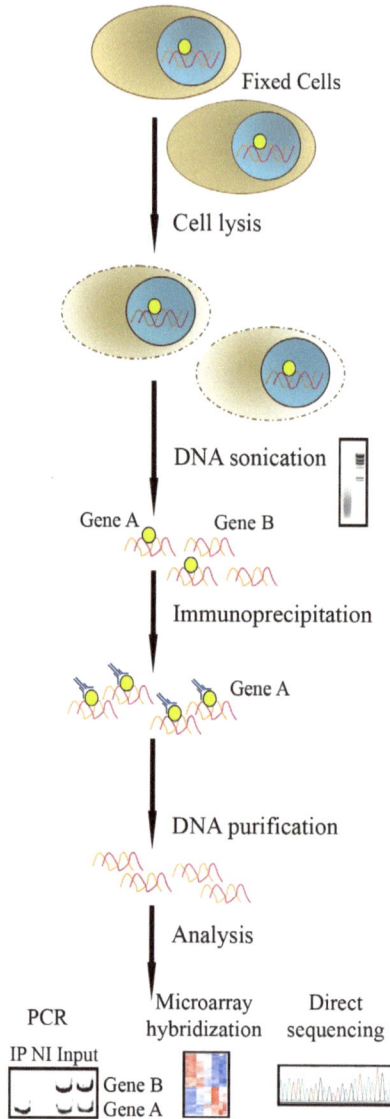

Figure 4: Outline of the chromatin immunoprecipitation (ChIP) procedure. Living cells or tissues are fixed with formaldehyde, thus covalently binding (crosslinking) amine groups placed in close proximity, such as those of the nitrogen bases in the DNA and the aminoacids in its associated proteins. Fixed cells are then lysed and the DNA is randomly sheared into small fragments by sonication or enzyme digestion. Sonicated DNA is then immunoprecipitated using an antibody against a particular transcription factor or modified histone. The DNA fragments thus selected are further purified and analyzed. The principal analysis methodologies employed include endpoint or real-time PCR using specific primers to detect the presence or absence of particular gene

sequences in the precipitated DNA, or global non-biased approaches such as microarray hybridization (ChIP-chip) or direct sequencing of the precipitated DNA using next generation technology (ChIP-Seq).

nucleolar RNAs (snoRNAs), all of which have relatively well-established functions in translation and splicing, the rest of ncRNAs were initially regarded as non-specific 'noise'. However, recent findings have unraveled a critical role for some of these RNA molecules in the regulation of gene expression and genomic stability. What these ncRNAs do and how they work is one of biology's contemporary hot topics. As research in this field continues to explode, one can anticipate that fascinating new insights on the function of these molecules will be uncovered in the years to come.

1.3.3.1. MicroRNAs and Piwi-Interacting RNAs

MicroRNAs (miRNAs) are one class of short ncRNAs of approximately 21 nucleotides in length that act as potent post-transcriptional regulators of the expression of genes. It has been predicted that the human genome may contain more than 1000 different miRNAs [103] that regulate at least 30% of all human genes [104]. Many of these miRNAs are conserved across species and display specific temporal and developmental expression patterns, in agreement with their evolutionarily conserved role in gene regulation. Indeed, miRNAs have been implicated in the control of a wide variety of biological processes ranging from proliferation and apoptosis to metabolism [105, 106].

MiRNAs are transcribed by RNA polymerase II from their own transcriptional units or, most frequently, are co-expressed from the intronic regions of their host genes [107]. Mature miRNAs are processed from partially folded stem-loop precursor RNAs by a two-step process involving the action of two different RNAse III enzymes, Drosha in the nucleus and Dicer in the cytoplasm [108, 109]. The generated mature single-stranded miRNA acts as a guide to ribonucleoprotein complexes (miRNP) that recognize complementary sequences in the 3'-untranslated regions (3'-UTR) of mRNAs. The mode of action of a particular miRNA highly depends on the degree of base complementarity with its target mRNA. If sequences are partially complementary, the miRNA represses mRNA translation. Conversely, if sequences are fully complementary, the miRNA leads to mRNA cleavage [110].

It is broadly acknowledged that epigenetics and microRNAs are intimately interconnected. On the one hand, the expression of miRNAs is under tight epigenetic control and loss of these epigenetic restraints has been associated to the etiology of several human cancers [111, 112]. On the other hand, miRNAs can control chromatin structure through the post-transcriptional regulation of key epigenetic remodelers [113]. This is best illustrated by a number of recent studies uncovering a direct link between miRNA function and the expression of DNMTs or histone modifying enzymes [114-116].

Another variety of small ncRNAs with ascribed roles in chromatin regulation are Piwi-interacting RNAs (piRNAs). These RNAs, of 21 to 30 nucleotides in length, are specifically expressed in testes and are needed for proper germ cell development. They are highly enriched in repetitive sequences and participate in the silencing of transposons during gametogenesis. This most likely occurs through regulation of *de novo* DNA methylation but the molecular mechanism involved remains to be elucidated [117, 118].

1.3.3.2. Large Intergenic Non-Coding RNAs

Mammalian cells express over a thousand evolutionarily conserved large intergenic non-coding transcripts known as lincRNAs [119]. Initially, these ncRNAs were thought to modulate expression of genes located in close proximity to the sites that produced them by interfering with specific DNA-bound transcription factors or with the basal transcriptional machinery [120]. However, in 2007, Rinn *et al.* provided the first evidence of how the lincRNA termed HOTAIR could affect expression of a gene at a distal location (a different chromosome) from the site encoding this ncRNA [121]. That surprising breakthrough led to the identification of an unexpected role for these RNAs in epigenetic regulation. Indeed, lincRNAs associate with repressive chromatin modifiers and assist in guiding these proteins to the proper locations in the genome [122-124]. In other words, they serve as modular scaffolds for epigenetic regulatory complexes in cells. Furthermore, recent findings have revealed that a transcription factor, p53, can regulate expression of many of these lincRNAs, which in turn regulate some of the p53 targetome [125]. These data, together with the fact that p53 is the most commonly mutated gene in cancer, strongly argue for a critical role of lincRNAs in cell development and gene regulation and, consequently, in human health and disease.

1.4. LIFESTYLE AND EPIGENETICS

Based on the increasing knowledge of how the complex epigenetic machinery can modulate gene expression patterns, it is now undisputed that the information stored in the genes is not limited to the inherited DNA sequence. One of the clearest examples to understand this phenomenon at the organismal level are the phenotypical and pathophysiological discordances that arise between monozygotic twin siblings during their lifetime, especially when they adopt different lifestyles and are exposed to dissimilar environments. It is now widely accepted that in most cases such divergence can be attributed to either stochastic, lifestyle or environmental factors that trigger modifications on top of the genetic information that was originally identical in the zygotes [126].

In the last few years, we have started to gain insight on the nature of the epigenetic mechanisms elicited by lifestyle and environment through studies in humans and animal models. For instance, it has been shown that exposure of rodents to an enriched environment that included cognitive, social, somatosensory, motor, and visual stimulating settings increased synaptic integrity and neuroplasticity in the brain, while improving memory, learning and stress response. Such effects correlated with changes in the acetylation and methylation of histones H3 and H4 in the hippocampus and cerebral cortex regions, starting within 3 hours of enriched environment exposure and some of them persisting for at least 2 weeks [127]. The practice of physical exercise also has a significant impact in the epigenome. In humans, it has recently been described that cycling induced a global increase in H3K36 acetylation and that the nuclear localization of HDAC4 and HDAC5 is reduced during exercise, indicating a decreased transcriptional repressive function [128]. In rats, physical exercise enhanced stress-coping abilities and this correlated with increased phosphoacetylation of histone H3 and c-Fos induction in dentate gyrus neurons [129]. Similarly, food bioactive components can strongly influence the epigenome through changes in specific enzymatic activities. For example, dietary factors found in cruciferous vegetables (*i.e.* sulforaphane and related isothiocyanates) exert anti-cancer effects through mechanisms including the inhibition of the activity of HDACs. Indeed, pilot studies in humans have shown HDAC inhibition in blood cells after consumption of a single dose of sulforaphane-rich broccoli sprouts [130]. Many other dietary phytochemicals have also been shown to interact with the epigenetic machinery and to influence the progression of diseases such as cancer, inflammatory diseases, neurodegenerative disorders, cardiovascular disease and obesity [131]. The social environment is another factor that can affect the epigenetic program. A seminal article showing how the epigenome of one subject can be influenced by the behavior of another is the study of epigenetic programming by maternal care by Meaney's group [132]. They showed that maternal behavior influenced the offspring's histone acetylation and DNA methylation status at the promoter of the glucocorticoid receptor gene in the hippocampus. These epigenetic modifications correlated with alterations of the stress response in the offspring. Interestingly, both the epigenetic and the behavioral impact of maternal care were reversed in adult offsprings by pharmacological treatment with the histone deacetylase inhibitor trichostatin A, demonstrating that although these changes are long-lasting, they are potentially reversible even in the adult. It remains to be determined whether lifestyle interventions such as social support and stress reduction practices during adult life can also modify the behavioral-dependent epigenetic programming. Although in many cases, the exact mechanisms responsible for the above mentioned processes are still unknown, the epigenetic modifiers activated in response to life experiences and environmental exposures are starting to be elucidated (Table 1).

Hence, through the prism of the now scientifically proven notion that lifestyle can modify the information encoded in our genome, we may soon see a transition towards a more participatory medicine in which a growing awareness of individual lifestyle choices will contribute to the prevention and treatment of illness.

ACKNOWLEDGEMENTS

The authors are indebted to the Spanish Ministry of Science and Innovation for funding (grants BFU2009-09988/BMC (MP), BFU2008-02299/BMC (RG) and SAF2010-15050 (PK)).

Table 1: List of some of the epigenetic modifiers activated in response to experience.

Enzyme	Activity	Mediates	References
Histone Acetyltransferases (HATs)			
Gcn5/PCAF Family			
PCAF	H3K9, H3K14, H3K18	Memory formation	[133, 134]
CBP/p300 family			
CBP/p300	-	epigallocatechin-3-gallate (green tea flavonoid) effects on inflammation	[135]
MYST family			
MYST1	H4K16	Chronic arsenic exposure (drinking water contaminant)	[136]
Histone Deacetylases (HDACs)			
Class I HDACs			
HDAC1	-	Response to psychostimulants	[137]
HDAC2	-	Memory formation	[138]
Class II HDACs			
HDAC4	-	Drug reinforcement Response to endurance exercise	[128, 139]
HDAC5	-	Chronic emotional stimuli Synaptic plasticity and memory Response to endurance exercise	[128, 140, 141]
Class III HADCs			
Sirt1	-	Synaptic plasticity, memory and cognition Caloric restriction-induced lifespan	[142-144]
Histone Methyltransferases (HMTs)			
SET Domain Lysine HMTs			
MLL	H3K4	Memory formation	[145]
SUV39H1	H3K9	Response to psychostimulants	[137]
G9a	H3K9	Cocaine-induced plasticity Adaptive behavior	[146, 147]
Histone Demethylases (HDMs)			
***Jumonji* Family Demethylases**			
JMJD2A	H3K9, H3K36	Long-term memory	[148]

Table 1: cont….

Phosphatases			
PP1	-	Long-term memory Drug addiction	[148, 149]
Kinases			
MSK1	H3S28	Drug addiction Memory formation	[150, 151]
DNA Methyltransferases (DNMTs)			
DNMT1	Maintenance methylation	Memory and learning Nutritional deficiency and brain development Response to cigarette smoking Asbestos fiber exposure	[152-156]
DNMT3A	*De novo* methylation	Memory and learning Response to cigarette smoking Drug sensitization	[152, 155, 157, 158]
DNMT3B	*De novo* methylation	Drug sensitization	[158]
Methyl Binding Proteins (MBDs)			
MeCP2	Methyl cytosine binding	Drug addiction Nutritional effect on brain development Early life stress and depression	[154, 159, 160-162]

REFERENCES

[1]   Tountas Y. The historical origins of the basic concepts of health promotion and education: the role of ancient Greek philosophy and medicine. Health Promot Int 2009; 24: 185-92.

[2]   Feuerstein G. The Yoga-Sutra of Patañjali: A New Translation and Commentary: Inner Traditions International. Rochester, Vermont 1989. (in Samadhi Pada, Sutras XXX-XXXII)

[3]   Lindstrom J, Louheranta A, Mannelin M, Rastas M, Salminen V, Eriksson J, *et al.* The Finnish Diabetes Prevention Study (DPS): Lifestyle intervention and 3-year results on diet and physical activity. Diabetes Care 2003; 26: 3230-6.

[4]   Li G, Zhang P, Wang J, Gregg EW, Yang W, Gong Q, *et al.* The long-term effect of lifestyle interventions to prevent diabetes in the China Da Qing Diabetes Prevention Study: a 20-year follow-up study. Lancet 2008; 371: 1783-9.

[5]   Goldberg RB, Temprosa M, Haffner S, Orchard TJ, Ratner RE, Fowler SE, *et al.* Effect of progression from impaired glucose tolerance to diabetes on cardiovascular risk factors and its amelioration by lifestyle and metformin intervention: the Diabetes Prevention Program randomized trial by the Diabetes Prevention Program Research Group. Diabetes Care 2009; 32: 726-32.

[6]   Rovio S, Kareholt I, Helkala EL, Viitanen M, Winblad B, Tuomilehto J, *et al.* Leisure-time physical activity at midlife and the risk of dementia and Alzheimer's disease. Lancet Neurol 2005; 4: 705-11.

[7]   Fordyce DE, Wehner JM. Physical activity enhances spatial learning performance with an associated alteration in hippocampal protein kinase C activity in C57BL/6 and DBA/2 mice. Brain Res 1993; 619: 111-9.

[8]   Gomez-Pinilla F, So V, Kesslak JP. Spatial learning and physical activity contribute to the induction of fibroblast growth factor: neural substrates for increased cognition associated with exercise. Neuroscience 1998; 85: 53-61.

[9]   van Praag H, Shubert T, Zhao C, Gage FH. Exercise enhances learning and hippocampal neurogenesis in aged mice. J Neurosci 2005; 25: 8680-5.

[10]   Narath E, Skalicky M, Viidik A. Voluntary and forced exercise influence the survival and body composition of ageing male rats differently. Exp Gerontol 2001; 36: 1699-711.

[11]   Kim YP, Kim H, Shin MS, Chang HK, Jang MH, Shin MC, *et al.* Age-dependence of the effect of treadmill exercise on cell proliferation in the dentate gyrus of rats. Neurosci Lett 2004; 355: 152-4.

[12]   Uysal N, Tugyan K, Kayatekin BM, Acikgoz O, Bagriyanik HA, Gonenc S, *et al.* The effects of regular aerobic exercise in adolescent period on hippocampal neuron density, apoptosis and spatial memory. Neurosci Lett 2005; 383: 241-5.

[13]   van Praag H, Kempermann G, Gage FH. Running increases cell proliferation and neurogenesis in the adult mouse dentate gyrus. Nat Neurosci 1999; 2: 266-70.

[14]   Farmer J, Zhao X, van Praag H, Wodtke K, Gage FH, Christie BR. Effects of voluntary exercise on synaptic plasticity and gene expression in the dentate gyrus of adult male Sprague-Dawley rats *in vivo*. Neuroscience 2004; 124: 71-9.

[15]   Garza AA, Ha TG, Garcia C, Chen MJ, Russo-Neustadt AA. Exercise, antidepressant treatment, and BDNF mRNA expression in the aging brain. Pharmacol Biochem Behav 2004; 77: 209-20.

[16]   Ross R, Bradshaw AJ. The future of obesity reduction: beyond weight loss. Nat Rev Endocrinol 2009; 5: 319-25.

[17]   Hunsberger JG, Newton SS, Bennett AH, Duman CH, Russell DS, Salton SR, *et al.* Antidepressant actions of the exercise-regulated gene VGF. Nat Med. 2007; 13: 1476-82.

[18]   Molteni R, Ying Z, Gomez-Pinilla F. Differential effects of acute and chronic exercise on plasticity-related genes in the rat hippocampus revealed by microarray. Eur J Neurosci 2002; 16: 1107-16.

[19]   Tong L, Shen H, Perreau VM, Balazs R, Cotman CW. Effects of exercise on gene-expression profile in the rat hippocampus. Neurobiol Dis 2001; 8: 1046-56.

[20]   Kim J, Lee HJ, Lee KW. Naturally occurring phytochemicals for the prevention of Alzheimer's disease. J Neurochem 2010; 112: 1415-30.

[21]   Haigis M, Sinclair D. Mammalian sirtuins: biological insights and disease relevance. Annu Rev Pathol 2010; 5: 253-95.

[22]   Shi Q, Shih CC, Lee KH. Novel anti-prostate cancer curcumin analogues that enhance androgen receptor degradation activity. Anticancer Agents Med Chem 2009; 9: 904-12.

[23]   Mann GE, Rowlands DJ, Li FY, de Winter P, Siow RC. Activation of endothelial nitric oxide synthase by dietary isoflavones: role of NO in Nrf2-mediated antioxidant gene expression. Cardiovasc Res 2007; 75: 261-74.

[24]   McEwen BS, Gianaros PJ. Central role of the brain in stress and adaptation: links to socioeconomic status, health, and disease. Ann N Y Acad Sci 2010; 1186: 190-222.

[25]   Watanabe Y, Weiland NG, McEwen BS. Effects of adrenal steroid manipulations and repeated restraint stress on dynorphin mRNA levels and excitatory amino acid receptor binding in hippocampus. Brain Res 1995; 680: 217-25.

[26]   Reagan LP, Rosell DR, Wood GE, Spedding M, Munoz C, Rothstein J, *et al*. Chronic restraint stress up-regulates GLT-1 mRNA and protein expression in the rat hippocampus: reversal by tianeptine. Proc Nat Acad Sci USA 2004; 101: 2179-84.

[27]   Wood GE, Young LT, Reagan LP, Chen B, McEwen BS. Stress-induced structural remodeling in hippocampus: prevention by lithium treatment. Proc Nat Acad Sci USA 2004; 101: 3973-8.

[28]   Benson H, Rosner BA, Marzetta BR, Klemchuk HM. Decreased blood-pressure in pharmacologically treated hypertensive patients who regularly elicited the relaxation response. Lancet 1974; 1: 289-91.

[29]   Ludwig DS, Kabat-Zinn J. Mindfulness in medicine. JAMA 2008; 300: 1350-2.

[30]   Dusek JA, Otu HH, Wohlhueter AL, Bhasin M, Zerbini LF, Joseph MG, *et al*. Genomic counter-stress changes induced by the relaxation response. PloS One 2008; 3: e2576.

[31]   Yang W, Omaye ST. Air pollutants, oxidative stress and human health. Mutat Res 2009; 674: 45-54.

[32]   Fakhrzadeh L, Laskin JD, Laskin DL. Ozone-induced production of nitric oxide and TNF-alpha and tissue injury are dependent on NF-kappaB p50. Am J Physiol Lung Cell Mol Physiol 2004; 287: L279-85.

[33]   Timblin C, BeruBe K, Churg A, Driscoll K, Gordon T, Hemenway D, *et al*. Ambient particulate matter causes activation of the c-jun kinase/stress-activated protein kinase cascade and DNA synthesis in lung epithelial cells. Cancer Res 1998; 58: 4543-7.

[34]   Nestler EJ. Review. Transcriptional mechanisms of addiction: role of DeltaFosB. Philos Trans R Soc Lon B Biol Sci 2008; 363: 3245-55.

[35]   Watson JD, Crick FH. Molecular structure of nucleic acids; a structure for deoxyribose nucleic acid. Nature 1953; 171: 737-8.

[36]   Watson JD, Crick FH. Genetical implications of the structure of deoxyribonucleic acid. Nature 1953; 171: 964-7.

[37]   Nirenberg M. Historical review: Deciphering the genetic code-a personal account. Trends Biochem Sci 2004; 29: 46-54.

[38]   Collins F. Has the revolution arrived? Nature 2010; 464: 674-5.

[39]   Venter JC. Multiple personal genomes await. Nature 2010 ;464:676-7.

[40]   Gibson DG, Glass JI, Lartigue C, Noskov VN, Chuang RY, Algire MA, *et al*. Creation of a bacterial cell controlled by a chemically synthesized genome. Science 2010; 329: 52-6.

[41]   Bernstein BE, Meissner A, Lander ES. The mammalian epigenome. Cell 2007; 128: 669-81.

[42]   Berger SL, Kouzarides T, Shiekhattar R, Shilatifard A. An operational definition of epigenetics. Genes Dev 2009; 23: 781-3.

[43]   Goldberg AD, Allis CD, Bernstein E. Epigenetics: a landscape takes shape. Cell. 2007; 128: 635-8.

[44]   D'Alessio AC, Szyf M. Epigenetic tete-a-tete: the bilateral relationship between chromatin modifications and DNA methylation. Biochem Cell Biol 2006; 84: 463-76.

[45]   Fuks F. DNA methylation and histone modifications: teaming up to silence genes. Curr Opin Genet Dev 2005; 15: 490-5.

[46]   Ehrlich M, Gama-Sosa MA, Huang LH, Midgett RM, Kuo KC, McCune RA, *et al*. Amount and distribution of 5-methylcytosine in human DNA from different types of tissues of cells. Nucleic Acids Res 1982; 10: 2709-21.

[47]   Ramsahoye BH, Biniszkiewicz D, Lyko F, Clark V, Bird AP, Jaenisch R. Non-CpG methylation is prevalent in embryonic stem cells and may be mediated by DNA methyltransferase 3a. Proc Nat Acad Sci USA 2000; 97: 5237-42.

[48]   Esteller M. Epigenetics in cancer. N Engl J Med 2008; 358: 1148-59.

[49]   Antequera F, Bird A. Number of CpG islands and genes in human and mouse. Proc Nat Acad Sci USA 1993; 90: 11995-9.

[50]   Walsh CP, Bestor TH. Cytosine methylation and mammalian development. Genes Dev 1999; 13: 26-34.

[51]   Li E, Bestor TH, Jaenisch R. Targeted mutation of the DNA methyltransferase gene results in embryonic lethality. Cell 1992; 69: 915-26.

[52]   Kaneda M, Okano M, Hata K, Sado T, Tsujimoto N, Li E, *et al.* Essential role for *de novo* DNA methyltransferase Dnmt3a in paternal and maternal imprinting. Nature 2004; 429: 900-3.

[53]   Goll MG, Kirpekar F, Maggert KA, Yoder JA, Hsieh CL, Zhang X, *et al.* Methylation of tRNAAsp by the DNA methyltransferase homolog Dnmt2. Science 2006; 311: 395-8.

[54]   Okano M, Xie S, Li E. Dnmt2 is not required for *de novo* and maintenance methylation of viral DNA in embryonic stem cells. Nucleic Acids Res 1998; 26: 2536-40.

[55]   Law JA, Jacobsen SE. Establishing, maintaining and modifying DNA methylation patterns in plants and animals. Nat Rev Gene. 2010; 11: 204-20.

[56]   Bourc'his D, Bestor TH. Meiotic catastrophe and retrotransposon reactivation in male germ cells lacking Dnmt3L. Nature 2004; 431: 96-9.

[57]   Hendrich B, Tweedie S. The methyl-CpG binding domain and the evolving role of DNA methylation in animals. Trends Genet 2003; 19: 269-77.

[58]   Fatemi M, Wade PA. MBD family proteins: reading the epigenetic code. J Cell Sci 2006; 119: 3033-7.

[59]   Goll MG, Bestor TH. Eukaryotic cytosine methyltransferases. Annu Rev Biochem 2005; 74: 481-514.

[60]   Morgan HD, Santos F, Green K, Dean W, Reik W. Epigenetic reprogramming in mammals. Hum Mol Genet 2005; 14: R47-58.

[61]   Kim MS, Kondo T, Takada I, Youn MY, Yamamoto Y, Takahashi S, *et al.* DNA demethylation in hormone-induced transcriptional derepression. Nature 2009; 461: 1007-12.

[62]   Wu H, Sun YE. Reversing DNA methylation: new insights from neuronal activity-induced Gadd45b in adult neurogenesis. Sci signal 2009; 2: pe17.

[63]   Zhu JK. Active DNA demethylation mediated by DNA glycosylases. Annu Rev Genet 2009; 43: 143-66.

[64]   Fraga MF, Esteller M. DNA methylation: a profile of methods and applications. BioTechniques 2002; 33:632.

[65]   Jacinto FV, Ballestar E, Esteller M. Methyl-DNA immunoprecipitation (MeDIP): hunting down the DNA methylome. BioTechniques 2008; 44: 35.

[66]   Ballestar E, Paz MF, Valle L, Wei S, Fraga MF, Espada J, *et al.* Methyl-CpG binding proteins identify novel sites of epigenetic inactivation in human cancer. EMBO J 2003; 22: 6335-45.

[67]   Weber M, Davies JJ, Wittig D, Oakeley EJ, Haase M, Lam WL, *et al.* Chromosome-wide and promoter-specific analyses identify sites of differential DNA methylation in normal and transformed human cells. Nat Genet 2005; 37: 853-62.

[68]   Couture JF, Trievel RC. Histone-modifying enzymes: encrypting an enigmatic epigenetic code. Curr Opin Struct Biol 2006; 16: 753-60.

[69]   Kouzarides T. Chromatin modifications and their function. Cell 2007; 128: 693-705.

[70]   Kristjuhan A, Walker J, Suka N, Grunstein M, Roberts D, Cairns BR, *et al.* Transcriptional inhibition of genes with severe histone H3 hypoacetylation in the coding region. Mol Cell 2002; 10: 925-33.

[71]   Kurdistani SK, Tavazoie S, Grunstein M. Mapping global histone acetylation patterns to gene expression. Cell 2004; 117: 721-33.

[72]   Bernstein BE, Humphrey EL, Erlich RL, Schneider R, Bouman P, Liu JS, *et al.* Methylation of histone H3 Lys 4 in coding regions of active genes. Proc Natl Acad Sci USA 2002; 99: 8695-700.

[73]   Santos-Rosa H, Schneider R, Bannister AJ, Sherriff J, Bernstein BE, Emre NC, *et al.* Active genes are tri-methylated at K4 of histone H3. Nature 2002; 419: 407-11.

[74]   Schneider R, Bannister AJ, Myers FA, Thorne AW, Crane-Robinson C, Kouzarides T. Histone H3 lysine 4 methylation patterns in higher eukaryotic genes. Nat Cell Biol 2004; 6: 73-7.

[75]   Lachner M, O'Carroll D, Rea S, Mechtler K, Jenuwein T. Methylation of histone H3 lysine 9 creates a binding site for HP1 proteins. Nature 2001; 410: 116-20.

[76]   Papp B, Muller J. Histone trimethylation and the maintenance of transcriptional ON and OFF states by trxG and PcG proteins. Genes Dev 2006; 20: 2041-54.

[77]   Jenuwein T, Allis CD. Translating the histone code. Science 2001; 293: 1074-80.

[78]   Agalioti T, Chen G, Thanos D. Deciphering the transcriptional histone acetylation code for a human gene. Cell 2002; 111: 381-92.

[79]   Deckert J, Struhl K. Histone acetylation at promoters is differentially affected by specific activators and repressors. Mol Cell Biol 2001; 21: 2726-35.

[80]   Katan-Khaykovich Y, Struhl K. Dynamics of global histone acetylation and deacetylation *in vivo*: rapid restoration of normal histone acetylation status upon removal of activators and repressors. Genes Dev 2002; 16: 743-52.

[81]   Kubicek S, Jenuwein T. A crack in histone lysine methylation. Cell 2004; 119: 903-6.

[82]   Klose RJ, Yamane K, Bae Y, Zhang D, Erdjument-Bromage H, Tempst P, *et al.* The transcriptional repressor JHDM3A demethylates trimethyl histone H3 lysine 9 and lysine 36. Nature. 2006; 442: 312-6.

[83]   Shi Y, Lan F, Matson C, Mulligan P, Whetstine JR, Cole PA, *et al.* Histone demethylation mediated by the nuclear amine oxidase homolog LSD1. Cell 2004; 119: 941-53.

[84]   Tsukada Y, Fang J, Erdjument-Bromage H, Warren ME, Borchers CH, Tempst P, *et al.* Histone demethylation by a family of JmjC domain-containing proteins. Nature 2006; 439: 811-6.

[85]   Whetstine JR, Nottke A, Lan F, Huarte M, Smolikov S, Chen Z, *et al.* Reversal of histone lysine trimethylation by the JMJD2 family of histone demethylases. Cell 2006; 125: 467-81.

[86]   Yamane K, Toumazou C, Tsukada Y, Erdjument-Bromage H, Tempst P, Wong J, *et al.* JHDM2A, a JmjC-containing H3K9 demethylase, facilitates transcription activation by androgen receptor. Cell 2006; 125: 483-95.

[87]   Shi YJ, Matson C, Lan F, Iwase S, Baba T, Shi Y. Regulation of LSD1 histone demethylase activity by its associated factors. Mol Cell 2005; 19: 857-64.

[88]   Wang J, Scully K, Zhu X, Cai L, Zhang J, Prefontaine GG, *et al.* Opposing LSD1 complexes function in developmental gene activation and repression programmes. Nature 2007; 446: 882-7.

[89]   Liang Y, Vogel JL, Narayanan A, Peng H, Kristie TM. Inhibition of the histone demethylase LSD1 blocks alpha-herpesvirus lytic replication and reactivation from latency. Nat Med 2009; 15: 1312-7.

[90]   Metzger E, Wissmann M, Yin N, Muller JM, Schneider R, Peters AH, *et al.* LSD1 demethylates repressive histone marks to promote androgen-receptor-dependent transcription. Nature 2005; 437: 436-9.

[91]   Klose RJ, Zhang Y. Regulation of histone methylation by demethylimination and demethylation. Nat Rev Mol Cell Biol 2007; 8: 307-18.

[92]   Tamaru H, Selker EU. A histone H3 methyltransferase controls DNA methylation in Neurospora crassa. Nature 2001; 414: 277-83.

[93]   Wang J, Hevi S, Kurash JK, Lei H, Gay F, Bajko J, *et al.* The lysine demethylase LSD1 (KDM1) is required for maintenance of global DNA methylation. Nat Genet 2009; 41: 125-9.

[94]   Epsztejn-Litman S, Feldman N, Abu-Remaileh M, Shufaro Y, Gerson A, Ueda J, *et al. De novo* DNA methylation promoted by G9a prevents reprogramming of embryonically silenced genes. Nat Str Mol Biol 2008; 15: 1176-83.

[95]   Dedon PC, Soults JA, Allis CD, Gorovsky MA. A simplified formaldehyde fixation and immunoprecipitation technique for studying protein-DNA interactions. Anal Biochem 1991; 197: 83-90.

[96]   Orlando V. Mapping chromosomal proteins *in vivo* by formaldehyde-crosslinked-chromatin immunoprecipitation. Trends Biochem Sci 2000; 25: 99-104.

[97]   Farnham PJ. Insights from genomic profiling of transcription factors. Nat Rev Genet 2009; 10: 605-16.

[98]   Park PJ. ChIP-seq: advantages and challenges of a maturing technology. Nat Rev Genet 2009; 10: 669-80.

[99]   Carninci P, Kasukawa T, Katayama S, Gough J, Frith MC, Maeda N, *et al.* The transcriptional landscape of the mammalian genome. Science 2005; 309: 1559-63.

[100] Frith MC, Pheasant M, Mattick JS. The amazing complexity of the human transcriptome. Eur J Hum Genet 2005; 13: 894-7.

[101] Kapranov P, Willingham AT, Gingeras TR. Genome-wide transcription and the implications for genomic organization. Nat Rev Genet 2007;8: 413-23.

[102] Birney E, Stamatoyannopoulos JA, Dutta A, Guigo R, Gingeras TR, Margulies EH, *et al.* Identification and analysis of functional elements in 1% of the human genome by the ENCODE pilot project. Nature 2007; 447: 799-816.

[103] Berezikov E, Guryev V, van de Belt J, Wienholds E, Plasterk RH, Cuppen E. Phylogenetic shadowing and computational identification of human microRNA genes. Cell 2005; 120: 21-4.

[104] Bartel DP. MicroRNAs: genomics, biogenesis, mechanism, and function. Cell 2004; 116:281-97.

[105] Krol J, Loedige I, Filipowicz W. The widespread regulation of microRNA biogenesis, function and decay. Nat Rev Genet 2010; 11: 597-610.

[106] Lynn FC, Skewes-Cox P, Kosaka Y, McManus MT, Harfe BD, German MS. MicroRNA expression is required for pancreatic islet cell genesis in the mouse. Diabetes 2007; 56: 2938-45.

[107] Kim VN, Nam JW. Genomics of microRNA. Trends Genet 2006; 22: 165-73.

[108] Lee Y, Jeon K, Lee JT, Kim S, Kim VN. MicroRNA maturation: stepwise processing and subcellular localization. EMBO J 2002; 21: 4663-70.

[109] Lee Y, Ahn C, Han J, Choi H, Kim J, Yim J, *et al.* The nuclear RNase III Drosha initiates microRNA processing. Nature 2003; 425: 415-9.

[110] Hutvagner G, Zamore PD. RNAi: nature abhors a double-strand. Curr Opin Genet Dev 2002; 12: 225-32.

[111] Melo SA, Esteller M. Dysregulation of microRNAs in cancer: Playing with fire. FEBSLett. 2010; in press

[112] van Wolfswinkel JC, Ketting RF. The role of small non-coding RNAs in genome stability and chromatin organization. J Cell Sci 2010; 123: 1825-39.

[113] Lewis BP, Burge CB, Bartel DP. Conserved seed pairing, often flanked by adenosines, indicates that thousands of human genes are microRNA targets. Cell 2005; 12: 15-20.

[114] Fabbri M, Garzon R, Cimmino A, Liu Z, Zanesi N, Callegari E, *et al.* MicroRNA-29 family reverts aberrant methylation in lung cancer by targeting DNA methyltransferases 3A and 3B. Proc Natl Acad Sci USA 2007; 104: 15805-10.

[115] Sinkkonen L, Hugenschmidt T, Berninger P, Gaidatzis D, Mohn F, Artus-Revel CG, *et al.* MicroRNAs control *de novo* DNA methylation through regulation of transcriptional repressors in mouse embryonic stem cells. Nat Struct Mol Biol 2008; 15: 259-67.

[116] Cao P, Deng Z, Wan M, Huang W, Cramer SD, Xu J, *et al.* MicroRNA-101 negatively regulates Ezh2 and its expression is modulated by androgen receptor and HIF-1alpha/HIF-1beta. Mol Cancer 2010; 9: 108.

[117] Aravin AA, Sachidanandam R, Girard A, Fejes-Toth K, Hannon GJ. Developmentally regulated piRNA clusters implicate MILI in transposon control. Science 2007; 316: 744-7.

[118] Carmell MA, Girard A, van de Kant HJ, Bourc'his D, Bestor TH, de Rooij DG, *et al.* MIWI2 is essential for spermatogenesis and repression of transposons in the mouse male germline. Dev Cell 2007; 12: 503-14.

[119] Guttman M, Amit I, Garber M, French C, Lin MF, Feldser D, *et al.* Chromatin signature reveals over a thousand highly conserved large non-coding RNAs in mammals. Nature 2009; 458: 223-7.

[120] Goodrich JA, Kugel JF. Non-coding-RNA regulators of RNA polymerase II transcription. Nat Rev Mol Cell Biol 2006; 7: 612-6.

[121] Rinn JL, Kertesz M, Wang JK, Squazzo SL, Xu X, Brugmann SA, *et al.* Functional demarcation of active and silent chromatin domains in human HOX loci by noncoding RNAs. Cell 2007; 129: 1311-23.

[122] Woo CJ, Kingston RE. HOTAIR lifts noncoding RNAs to new levels. Cell 2007; 129: 1257-9.

[123] Khalil AM, Guttman M, Huarte M, Garber M, Raj A, Rivea Morales D, *et al.* Many human large intergenic noncoding RNAs associate with chromatin-modifying complexes and affect gene expression. Proc Nat Acad Sci USA 2009; 106: 11667-72.

[124] Tsai MC, Manor O, Wan Y, Mosammaparast N, Wang JK, Lan F, *et al.* Long noncoding RNA as modular scaffold of histone modification complexes. Science 2010; 329: 689-93.

[125] Huarte M, Guttman M, Feldser D, Garber M, Koziol MJ, Kenzelmann-Broz D, *et al.* A large intergenic noncoding RNA induced by p53 mediates global gene repression in the p53 response. Cell 2010; 142: 409-19.

[126] Poulsen P, Esteller M, Vaag A, Fraga MF. The epigenetic basis of twin discordance in age-related diseases. Pediatr Res 2007; 61: 38R-42R.

[127] Fischer A, Sananbenesi F, Wang X, Dobbin M, Tsai LH. Recovery of learning and memory is associated with chromatin remodelling. Nature 2007; 447: 178-82.

[128] McGee SL, Fairlie E, Garnham AP, Hargreaves M. Exercise-induced histone modifications in human skeletal muscle. J Physiol 2009; 587: 5951-8.

[129] Collins A, Hill LE, Chandramohan Y, Whitcomb D, Droste SK, Reul JM. Exercise improves cognitive responses to psychological stress through enhancement of epigenetic mechanisms and gene expression in the dentate gyrus. PloS One 2009; 4: e4330.

[130] Dashwood RH, Ho E. Dietary agents as histone deacetylase inhibitors: sulforaphane and structurally related isothiocyanates. Nutr Rev 2008; 66: S36-8.

[131] Szarc Vel Szic K, Ndlovu MN, Haegeman G, Vanden Berghe W. Nature or nurture: Let food be your epigenetic medicine in chronic inflammatory disorders. Biochem Pharmacol 2010; in press

[132] Weaver IC, Cervoni N, Champagne FA, D'Alessio AC, Sharma S, Seckl JR, *et al.* Epigenetic programming by maternal behavior. Nat Neurosci 2004; 7: 847-54.

[133] Duclot F, Jacquet C, Gongora C, Maurice T. Alteration of working memory but not in anxiety or stress response in p300/CBP associated factor (PCAF) histone acetylase knockout mice bred on a C57BL/6 background. Neurosci Lett 2010; 475: 179-83.

[134] Maurice T, Duclot F, Meunier J, Naert G, Givalois L, Meffre J, *et al.* Altered memory capacities and response to stress in p300/CBP-associated factor (PCAF) histone acetylase knockout mice. Neuropsychopharmacology 2008; 33: 1584-602.

[135] Choi KC, Jung MG, Lee YH, Yoon JC, Kwon SH, Kang HB *et al.* Epigallocatechin-3-gallate, a histone acetyltransferase inhibitor, inhibits EBV-induced B lymphocyte transformation *via* suppression of RelA acetylation. Cancer Res 2009;69: 583-92.

[136] Jo WJ, Ren X, Chu F, Aleshin M, Wintz H, Burlingame A *et al.* Acetylated H4K16 by MYST1 protects UROtsa cells from arsenic toxicity and is decreased following chronic arsenic exposure.Toxicol Appl Pharmacol 2009; 241: 294-302.

[137] Renthal W, Nestler EJ. Epigenetic mechanisms in drug addiction. Trends Mol Med 2008; 14: 341-50.

[138] Guan JS, Haggarty SJ, Giacometti E, Dannenberg JH, Joseph N, Gao J, *et al.* HDAC2 negatively regulates memory formation and synaptic plasticity. Nature 2009; 459: 55-60.

[139] Wang L, Lv Z, Hu Z, Sheng J, Hui B, Sun J, *et al.* Chronic cocaine-induced H3 acetylation and transcriptional activation of CaMKIIalpha in the nucleus accumbens is critical for motivation for drug reinforcement. Neuropsychopharmacology 2010; 35: 913-28.

[140] Renthal W, Maze I, Krishnan V, Covington HE, III, Xiao G, Kumar A, *et al.* Histone deacetylase 5 epigenetically controls behavioral adaptations to chronic emotional stimuli. Neuron 2007; 56: 517-29.

[141] Guan Z, Giustetto M, Lomvardas S, Kim JH, Miniaci MC, Schwartz JH, *et al.* Integration of long-term-memory-related synaptic plasticity involves bidirectional regulation of gene expression and chromatin structure. Cell 2002;111: 483-93

[142] Gao J, Wang WY, Mao YW, Graff J, Guan JS, Pan L, *et al.* A novel pathway regulates memory and plasticity *via* SIRT1 and miR-134. Nature 2010; 466: 1105-9.

[143] Michan S, Li Y, Chou MM, Parrella E, Ge H, Long JM, *et al.* SIRT1 is essential for normal cognitive function and synaptic plasticity. J Neurosci 2010; 30: 9695-707.

[144] Wood JG, Rogina B, Lavu S, Howitz K, Helfand SL, Tatar M, *et al.* Sirtuin activators mimic caloric restriction and delay ageing in metazoans. Nature 2004; 430: 686-9.

[145] Gupta S, Kim SY, Artis S, Molfese DL, Schumacher A, Sweatt JD, *et al.* Histone methylation regulates memory formation. J Neurosci 2010; 30: 3589-99.

[146] Maze I, Covington HE, III, Dietz DM, LaPlant Q, Renthal W, Russo SJ, *et al.* Essential role of the histone methyltransferase G9a in cocaine-induced plasticity. Science 2010; 327: 213-6.

[147] Schaefer A, Sampath SC, Intrator A, Min A, Gertler TS, Surmeier DJ, *et al.* Control of cognition and adaptive behavior by the GLP/G9a epigenetic suppressor complex. Neuron 2009; 64: 678-91.

[148] Koshibu K, Graff J, Beullens M, Heitz FD, Berchtold D, Russig H, *et al.* Protein phosphatase 1 regulates the histone code for long-term memory. J Neurosci 2009; 29: 13079-89.

[149] Gong JP, Liu QR, Zhang PW, Wang Y, Uhl GR. Mouse brain localization of the protein kinase C-enhanced phosphatase 1 inhibitor KEPI (kinase C-enhanced PP1 inhibitor). Neuroscience 2005; 132: 713-27.

[150] Brami-Cherrier K, Roze E, Girault JA, Betuing S, Caboche J. Role of the ERK/MSK1 signalling pathway in chromatin remodelling and brain responses to drugs of abuse. J Neurochem 2009; 108: 1323-35.

[151] Chwang WB, Arthur JS, Schumacher A, Sweatt JD. The nuclear kinase mitogen- and stress-activated protein kinase 1 regulates hippocampal chromatin remodeling in memory formation. J Neurosci 2007; 27: 12732-42.

[152] Feng J, Zhou Y, Campbell SL, Le T, Li E, Sweatt JD, *et al.* Dnmt1 and Dnmt3a maintain DNA methylation and regulate synaptic function in adult forebrain neurons. Nat Neurosci 2010; 13: 423-30.

[153] Kovacheva VP, Mellott TJ, Davison JM, Wagner N, Lopez-Coviella I, Schnitzler AC, *et al.* Gestational choline deficiency causes global and Igf2 gene DNA hypermethylation by up-regulation of Dnmt1 expression. J Biol Chem 2007; 282: 31777-88.

[154] Ke X, Lei Q, James SJ, Kelleher SL, Melnyk S, Jernigan S, *et al.* Uteroplacental insufficiency affects epigenetic determinants of chromatin structure in brains of neonatal and juvenile IUGR rats. Physiol Genomics 2006; 25: 16-28.

[155] Liu F, Killian JK, Yang M, Walker RL, Hong JA, Zhang M, *et al.* Epigenomic alterations and gene expression profiles in respiratory epithelia exposed to cigarette smoke condensate. Oncogene 2010; 29: 3650-64.

[156] Amatori S, Papalini F, Lazzarini R, Donati B, Bagaloni I, Rippo MR, *et al.* Decitabine, differently from DNMT1 silencing, exerts its antiproliferative activity through p21 upregulation in malignant pleural mesothelioma (MPM) cells. Lung Cancer 2009; 66:184-90.

[157] Liu H, Zhou Y, Boggs SE, Belinsky SA, Liu J. Cigarette smoke induces demethylation of prometastatic oncogene synuclein-gamma in lung cancer cells by downregulation of DNMT3B. Oncogene 2007; 26: 5900-10.

[158] Anier K, Malinovskaja K, Aonurm-Helm A, Zharkovsky A, Kalda A. DNA Methylation Regulates Cocaine-Induced Behavioral Sensitization in Mice. Neuropsychopharmacology 2010; 35: 2450-61.

[159] Deng JV, Rodriguiz RM, Hutchinson AN, Kim IH, Wetsel WC, West AE. MeCP2 in the nucleus accumbens contributes to neural and behavioral responses to psychostimulants. Nat Neurosci 2010; 13: 1128-36.

[160] Im HI, Hollander JA, Bali P, Kenny PJ. MeCP2 controls BDNF expression and cocaine intake through homeostatic interactions with microRNA-212. Nat Neurosci 2010; 13: 1120-7.

[161] Murgatroyd C, Patchev AV, Wu Y, Micale V, Bockmuhl Y, Fischer D, *et al.* Dynamic DNA methylation programs persistent adverse effects of early-life stress. Nat Neurosci 2009; 12: 1559-66.

[162] Murgatroyd C, Wu Y, Bockmuhl Y, Spengler D. Genes learn from stress: How infantile trauma programs us for depression. Epigenetics 2010; 5: 194 -9

CHAPTER 2

Epigenetics of Memory: Evidence and Models

Bechara J. Saab[*] and Isabelle M. Mansuy

Brain Research Institute, University of Zürich and Swiss Federal Institute of Technology, Zürich, Switzerland

Abstract: There is strong evidence that the epigenetic regulation of gene transcription, by way of covalent modifications of DNA and DNA-associated proteins, and through microRNAs, is an essential process underlying neuronal plasticity and memory. This chapter brings the non-specialist reader up to speed on important concepts within memory research, focusing on the role of the hippocampus, the molecular regulation of synaptic strength, and the behavioral tools used to examine learning and memory in experimental animals. Next, we describe the close association that is observed between defective epigentic processes and impaired memory in several cognitive diseases. The bulk of the chapter is then devoted to describing three broad classes of technical approaches that have been used to better understand how DNA methylation, histone post-translational modification, and microRNAs might contribute to memory. We end the chapter with a discussion on the potential relevance of epigenetic processes in sustaining memory traces in the brain over very long periods of time.

Keywords: Epigenetics, memory, plasticity, hippocampus, DNA methylation, histone code, microRNA.

2.1. INTRODUCTION

2.1.1. The Case for Epigenetic Encoding of Memory

The regulation of gene expression is a major mechanism through which cellular characteristics are set and altered. Currently, there are three widely recognized modes of epigenetic regulation: 1) the covalent modification of DNA itself; 2) the covalent modification of histone proteins that control the packaging of DNA into chromatin; and 3) small non-coding RNAs such as microRNAs that control messenger RNAs (mRNAs) and their translation into proteins. Since all three mechanisms modulate protein synthesis at some level, and since the synthesis of new proteins is required for long-term memory [1], processes of epigenetics likely underlie at least some aspects of memory.

[*]**Address correspondence to Bechara J. Saab:** Brain Research Institute, University of Zürich and Swiss Federal Institute of Technology, Winterthurerstrasse 190, CH-8057 Zürich, Switzerland; Tel: +41 44 635 33 64; Fax: +41 44 635 33 03; E-mail: saab@hifo.uzh.ch

Marcelina Párrizas, Rosa Gasa and Perla Kaliman (Eds)

The theory that DNA is a template upon which neurons etch a memory trace [2] emerged almost immediately following the discovery that transcription of DNA is essential to long-term memory [1]. In 1969, Griffith and Mahler proposed that "the physical basis of memory could lie in the enzymatic modifications of the DNA of nerve cells," thereby suggesting a direct role of epigenetics in memory storage. They reasoned that perhaps "the peculiarity that nerve cells possess of not dividing (exists) so as to avoid disturbing the learned information which is somehow stored in their DNA." Of course, division of a neuron would not only disturb the "learned information" on DNA, but would also upset the structure of neurons, and the positions of their synapses in the highly-organised, yet dynamic central nervous system. Nevertheless, although the precise "DNA Ticketing Theory," simultaneously proposed by Griffith and Mahler to potentially underlie memory [2] does not seem to occur, Griffith and Mahler were correct in the sense that neurons likely use epigenetic mechanisms as a means to control transcriptional events critical for the establishment and maintenance of memory.

The idea that the covalent modification of DNA might play a role in memory formation and storage was reintroduced by Francis Crick in 1984 [3], and further refined by Robin Holliday in 1999 [4] with the specific statement that "the exceptional stability required (for long-term memory) suggests…essential memory components may be based on…the enzymatic modification of cytosine in DNA to 5-methyl cytosine". Holliday reasoned that, due to the long-lasting nature of memory and the long-lasting effects on gene transcription that can result from a single DNA methylation event, it was reasonable to suspect neurons might capitalize on DNA methylation as a mechanism to maintain memory. His theorized that a singular event change in the DNA of a neuron might be coupled to the firing of that neuron following a specific stimulus, such that the specific stimulus would then be forever "remembered" by that cell in the form of a DNA methylation event. While difficult to either comprehensively prove or disprove at this point in time, there also exist alternative concepts for how memories might be formed and stored that do not require the persistence of any specific covalent biochemical events within neurons, on DNA or otherwise [5]. All theories of memory do however rely on synaptic transmission between neurons. For this reason, and because of their potential to act locally at individual synapses [6], microRNAs may play a central role in the fine-tuned set-up and maintenance of memory.

This chapter, published at a time when an epigenetic contribution to memory is just becoming a well-accepted concept, examines the current evidence. Recent advances in understanding the role of epigenetics in the maintenance of long-term memory are described in several sections, each introducing various experimental techniques. We then provide a simple model for how epigenetic events might act in concert to control plasticity and memory formation. We end by discussing the potential future of epigenetic research with respect to memory formation and provide the reader with some reserved predictions on how understanding the role of epigenetics in memory might refine our understanding of the brain.

2.1.2. Synaptic Plasticity and Neuronal Encoding of Memory

The encoding, storage and recall of memory are arguably the most fundamental aspects of a cognitive being. Many memories appear stable close to the entire lifetime of a human, and the same is true in widely used experimental animal models [7, 8]. The role of the mammalian hippocampus in establishing long-term memory was first demonstrated by accident, and in a dramatic fashion, when it and neighboring regions of an epileptic patient were removed to subdue frequent and severe seizures [9-11]. Patient Henry Molaison was left without any ability to form new autobiographical memory, and in a sense, for him time stopped. The relationship between the formation of long-term memory and an intact, functional hippocampus has since been substantiated many times in directed experiments with animals [11-16].

Synthesis of new products within the hippocampus during and soon after a learning event is essential for the transition of short-term spatial memory to long-term memory [17-20]. Several proteins as well as non-coding RNAs have been shown to be the targets of this synthesis, and nearly all of these are involved in synaptic transmission. The observation that transcriptional products underlying the strength of synaptic transmission are necessary for long-term memory formation, supports a much older theory stating that changes in synaptic efficacy are fundamental to the encoding of memory [21].

Long-term potentiation (LTP), a form of long-lasting synaptic plasticity found in the mammalian brain [22, 23], is strongly correlated with learning and memory. Inbred strains of mice with the highest hippocampal LTP also show the best spatial learning and memory [24]. Likewise, facilitation of LTP by genetic manipulations in mice has been associated with improved learning and memory (for excellent examples, see refs. [15, 25, 26]; for a review, see ref. [27]), while the disruption of LTP impairs learning and memory (for example, see ref. [28]). Finally, LTP occurs in the hippocampus during learning [29].

LTP, translation, transcription and synaptic specificity are all integral to learning, but how memory is actually stored in the brain is still a question of debate. Some argue memory is stored as a chemical event, potentially on DNA, or localized to a single synapse. Others believe memory is maintained as an electrical engram of persistent neuronal activity, whereby a circuit will fire asynchronously and in a stable manner, serving as a continued representation of information in the absence of the information's continued availability to the sensory system. In the final sections of this chapter, and in Box 1, we integrate recent advances in epigenetics into a framework in which molecular events (molecular memory traces) allow for and help stabilize persistence neuronal activity (electrical memory engrams), as a means to store memory in the brain.

The mouse hippocampus (see Fig. **1**) contains three main subregions: the dentate gyrus, and areas CA1 and CA3, and each are believed to underly distinct, separate processes in memory formation. The dentate gyrus receives the major innervation of excitatory transmission to the hippocampus, most of which originates in layers two and three of the entorhinal cortex [30, 31]. Dentate gyrus granule neurons, in turn, send axons to area CA3 and form synapses primarily onto pyramidal cells. The major collaterals leaving area CA3 then project around the inside arm of the dentate gyrus, innervate area CA1 and form synapses with dendrites on pyramidal neurons in area CA1. Finally, CA1 afferents complete the circuit through their synaptic connections in the entorhinal cortex, while simultaneously branching out to other cortical areas. All together, this circuitry is known as the trisynaptic hippocampal loop (Fig. **1**) and its very organization provides insight into the processing of information from the external world. For example, there are ten times as many cortical neurons sending axons onto a single granule cell in the dentate gyrus, than there are dentate gyrus granule cells contacting a single CA3 pyramidal cell. This pronounced imbalance in cellular interconnectivity may be needed to simplify neuronal firing patterns generated by complex sensory experiences. Reducing the number of cells communicating with an individual CA3 cell could be used to filter out less salient stimuli. In this way, only the information used for a memory can fully pass through the dentate gyrus and onto area CA3. In turn, changing the threshold of the filter could alter the robustness to form new memories, a possibility that may explain why selective enhancement of plasticity at cortico-dentate synapses increases the speed and ability of spatial learning [15]. Enhanced cortico-dentate plasticity therefore, may allow neurons of the dentate gyrus to more readily encode aspects of the outside world.

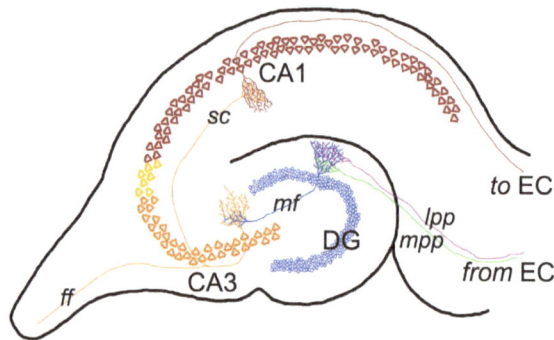

Figure 1: The hippocampal trisynaptic loop. Afferents from the entorhinal cortex (EC) innervate the dentate gyrus (DG) *via* the lateral and medial perforant paths (llp; mpp). From the DG, mossy fibers (mf) synapse onto pyramidal cells in area CA3. From area CA3, the Schaffer collateral (sc) axonal path contacts pyramidal cells in area CA1. Finally, neurons in area CA1 project back to the EC, completing the loop. Area CA3 also extends afferents *via* the fimbria fornix (ff) to extrahippocampal structures. Only the major and excitatory synaptic connections are shown.

Most glutamatergic synapses within the hippocampus contain two main types of glutamate-activated receptors, α-amino-3-hydroxy-5-methyl-4-isoxazolepropionic acid receptors (AMPARs) and N-methyl-D-aspartate receptors (NMDAR) (see Fig. **2**). Glutamate-bound AMPARs are permeable to sodium and mediate the majority of synaptic current in adult neurons. NMDARs, activated by the simultaneous binding of both glutamate and a co-agonist [32] are permeable to both sodium and calcium, and are essential for synaptic plasticity [33]. NMDARs also require membrane depolarization to open and therefore can act as a coincidence detector [34]. Blockade of NMDARs by pharmacological antagonists for instance, prevents LTP in area CA1 [33] and in the dentate gyrus [35, 36]. Likewise, inhibiting NMDARs or preventing calcium influx through the receptors

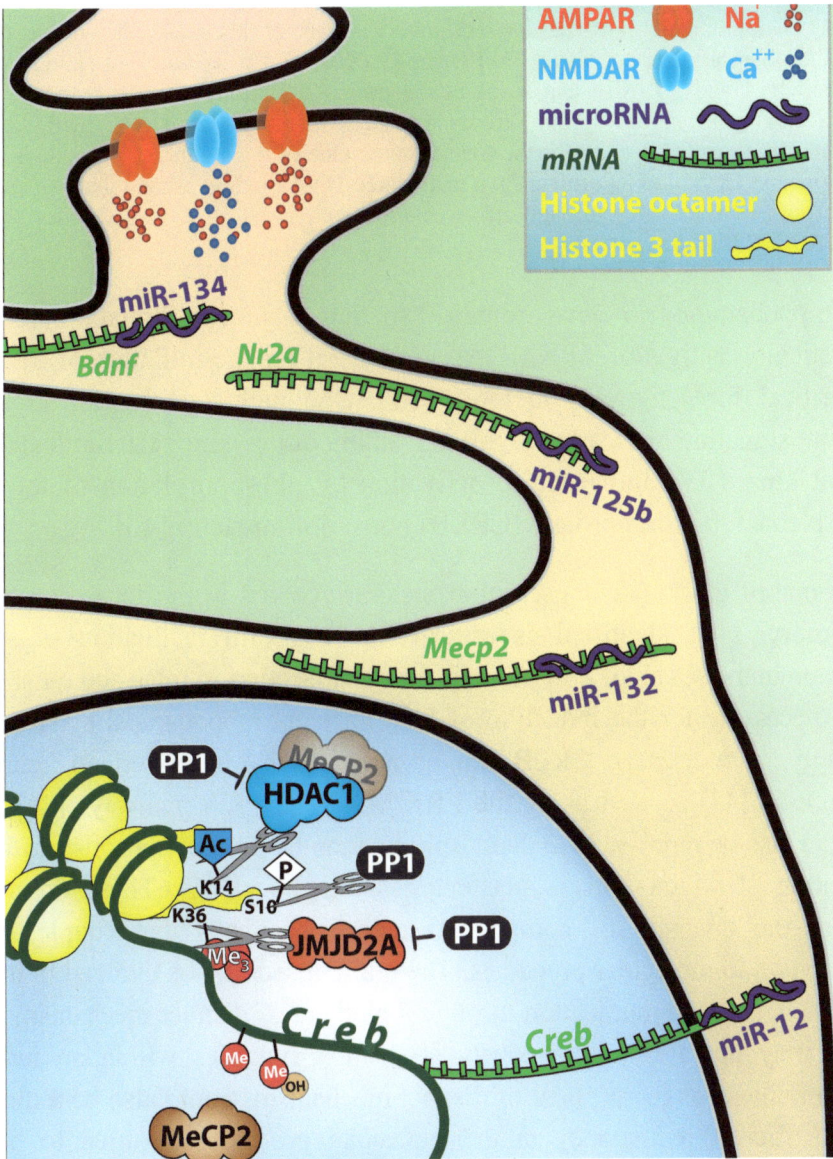

Figure 2: Epigenetic regulation of transcription and translation potentially underlying synaptic plasticity. In this neuronal model, Na$^+$ influx through AMPARs followed by Ca^{++} influx through NMDARs triggers a signaling cascade (not represented) that can activate or repress the action of microRNAs in the cell soma (cytosol), or locally in dendritic spines or axon terminals. As examples, relief of the action of miR-134 could allow for local synaptic production of BDNF and long-lasting facilitation of synaptic strength, while relief of the action of miR-125b could modify the level of the NMDAR subunit NR2A and alter glutamatergic neurotransmission. In the nucleus, protein phosphatase 1 (PP1) can be activated or repressed and influence chromatin modifying

enzymes such as HDAC1 (histone deacetylase 1) and JMJD2A (jumonji domain-containing protein 2A) that modulate post-translational modifications of histones. Shown are the PP1-regulated phosphorylation (P) of histone 3 at serine 10 (S10), and acetylation (Ac) and methylation (Me) of lysine 14 and 36 (K14 and K36) at the promoter of *Creb* (cAMP response element binding), a key gene in the formation of long-term memory. On DNA, methylation and hydroxymethylation can also control gene transcription. One of the mediators of methylated DNA is MeCP2 (methyl CpG binding protein 2), a methylated-DNA binding protein that can act as both a gene repressor and activator through an association with HDAC1. *Creb* is transcribed in the absence of MeCP2 binding.

in the hippocampus *in vivo* impairs spatial memory formation [37, 38]. Mechanistically, activation of NMDARs is critical for the initiation of translation events critical for long-term memory [39]. One pathway recruits a calcium-dependent signaling cascade involving calmodulin and calcium/calmodulin dependent kinase IV, and leads to activation by phosphorylation of the cAMP response element binding protein (CREB) transcription factor [40].

CREB is one of the major transcription factors involved in the formation of long-term memory. First identified as critical for long-term facilitation of synaptic transmission in the sea slug, *Aplysia* [41], follow up studies in mice and rat show that it is also necessary for the induction of LTP at many hippocampal synapses [42]. Interestingly, in mammals, CREB can be activated by brain-derived neurotropic factor (BDNF) [43] as well as by the ERK/MAP and PKA pathways [44]. CREB activity can also be repressed *via* dephosphorylation by protein phosphatase 1 (PP1), augmentation of which impairs plasticity and memory [45]. These observations underscore the diversity of components and mechanisms that couple synaptic communication to molecular processes. The brain, it seems, has evolved to maintain and change neural communication through a plethora of distinct mechanisms, many of which may operate simultaneously at distinct synapses within an individual neuron. Simultaneous recruitment of distinct mechanisms could also be a means for ensuring sufficient redundancy in the molecular processes required to maintain memory, a concept to which we return later.

2.1.3. Behavioral Paradigms for the Study of Memory in Rodents

In rodents, a number of behavioral tasks have been developed to study learning and memory. Tasks that depend on spatial abilities are ideal to assess hippocampal function, since the hippocampus is recruited for the processing of polymodal information of perception.

A number of behavioral tasks have thus been developed to examine spatially-dependent forms of associative memory. Conditioned place preference is a test based on the conditioning of an animal to one place over another. If a mouse or a rat is systematically injected with a rewarding substance, such as cocaine, in one environment, and with saline in another environment, the animal will demonstrate over time a preference for the drug-associated environment when given a choice between the two [46, 47]. The reverse can also be achieved with contextual fear conditioning, in which an animal learns to associate a given environment with a mild electric shock. When returned to the shock-associated context, mice demonstrate fear by adopting a characteristic motionless stature, termed freezing [48]. In the water maze test, a more complex task assessing spatial memory, rodents are placed in a pool of opaque water and have to navigate to an escape platform positioned just below the water surface (and thus invisible) [49]. In all of the many hippocampus-dependent versions of the water maze task, subjects are required to use distal spatial cues to navigate to the platform location, and escape from the pool [50].

Capitalizing on the innate curiosity of animals, object exploration in an experimental arena can also be used to assess memory based on novelty. Compared to familiar stimuli, both mice and rats more thoroughly explore objects to which they have never before been exposed [51]. Importantly, even placing a familiar object in a novel location within a given environment is sufficient to induce and increase exploration of that object compared to familiar objects that remain stationary [52]. The recognition of displacement can be designed so that, like the water maze, it depends on distal spatial cues and thus recruits the hippocampus. However, it is still debated whether novel object recognition (without displacement) is also hippocampus-dependent. Together, these paradigms (as well as others not described here) provide experimenters with powerful instruments to evaluate memory in rodents, and are therefore indispensible for memory research.

2.2. SUPPORT FOR EPIGENETICS IN MEMORY

2.2.1. Association with Cognitive Disorders

One major clue that epigenetic mechanisms have a role in learning and memory stems from the observation that disruption of epigenetic processes is often associated with cognitive disorders [53]. Epigenetic dysregulation has been reported in Rubinstein-Taybi syndrome, Rett syndrome, Fragile X syndrome, Alzheimer's disease, Huntington's disease, and schizophrenia; and all these illnesses affect learning and memory. In animal models of human disease, the study of endophenotypes (quantifiable symptoms of a disease with a defined biological origin) allows for an understanding of the molecular processes underlying specific symptoms of the disease [54].

In the rare congenital Rubinstein–Taybi syndrome (also known as Broad thumbhallux syndrome), the hallmark features of stunted stature, skeletal abnormality, and modest-to-severe mental retardation, could be due, at least in part, to perturbed epigenetic regulation in neurons. Most patients with this syndrome carry mutations in CREB binding protein (CBP) [55], a binding partner of the transcription factor CREB that, as already discussed, is known to be involved in memory formation [41, 56]. CBP has intrinsic histone acetyltransferase (HAT) activity [57] and is also critical for long-term memory [58], indicating the potential importance of regulating histone post-translational modifications (PTMs) during the formation of memory. Specific disruption of the HAT activity of CPB in mice leads to cognitive impairments characteristic of the Rubinstein-Taybi syndrome [59]. In human, the specific loss of CBP HAT activity also results in Rubinstein-Taybi syndrome [60-62]. Finally, defects in CPB are, as expected, associated with abnormal expression of CBP-regulated genes, including those downstream of CREB [61]. Overall, the molecular basis of cognitive alterations in Rubinstein-Taybi syndrome supports the idea that epigenetic mechanisms related to histone modifications are critical to the processes of learning and memory.

Rett syndrome, a more common congenital disorder than Rubinstein-Taybi syndrome, is similarly characterized by growth defects and modest-to-severe mental retardation, but unlike Rubinstein-Taybi syndrome, Rett syndrome can also be accompanied by microcephaly [63]. The symptoms of Rett syndrome are often caused by mutations in methyl-CpG binding protein 2 (MeCP2) [64], and the disease is well-modeled in mice lacking the *Mecp2* gene [65, 66]. Of particular relevance to epigenetics, MeCP2 transcriptionally represses genes containing methylated CpG islands, and serves to condense chromatin through a direct interaction with histones [67]. Interestingly, and we will return again to this concept, MeCP2 directly interacts with histone deacetylases (HDACs) in the mediation of chromatin remodeling [68], demonstrating the tight link that exists between DNA methylation and histone modification. Expression of MeCP2 is controlled by the microRNA, miR-132 and overexpression of miR-132 in mouse forebrain impairs learning, thereby modeling some of the cognitive phenotypes of the disorder [69]. Moreover, the onset of Rett syndrome endophenotypes in mice lacking the *Mecp2* gene is accompanied by dysregulation of a number of microRNAs [70, 71], including several that likely target BDNF [70]. The association of MeCP2 and Rett syndrome, with connection to three separate epigenetic mechanisms, suggests epigenetics play a general role in cognitive functions.

Fragile X syndrome is another relatively common heritable, congenital disease associated with mental retardation and also linked to epigenetic dysregulation. Erroneous expansion of trinucleotide repeats in the genes encoding fragile X mental retardation proteins 1 and 2 (FMR1 and FMR2, collectively as FMRPs) is associated with increased transcriptional repression of FMR1 and FMR2, through altered DNA methylation, and is believed to underlie the disorder [72-74]. In the mouse brain, FMR1 associates with several microRNAs, including miR-132 [75] that, as just mentioned, targets MeCP2 [69]. Further, microRNAs have been shown to control the transcription of FMRPs [76]. More research is needed to investigate the role of epigenetics in Fragile X syndrome, but since FMR1 binds ribonucleic acids directly, a prominent role for microRNAs in the disease is likely. FMR1 also interacts directly with Dicer, an important component of the microRNA processing machinery [77] (see Chapter 1).

While serving as an illustrative example for a role of epigenetics in cognitive functions, the association between epigenetic mechanisms and mental retardation provide little mechanistic insight into how epigenetics might regulate memory in the healthy brain. Further, developmental abnormalities in these disorders (potentially also caused by epigenetic dysregulation) could indirectly perturb processes needed to establish and maintain memory.

Alzheimer's disease (AD) is also associated with cognitive impairments, but unlike the three previous examples, is late-onset, neurodegenerative, and very common, affecting over 20 million people worldwide [78]. Unlike the congenial disorders already discussed, AD is not associated with any physical anomalies, and is often un-noticed until late stages of the disease. In some familial forms of AD, mutations in presenilin 1 (PS1) prevent PS1-dependent degradation of CBP, resulting in an up-regulation of CREB-dependent transcription [79]. Intriguingly, hypomethylation of the PS1 promoter region increases gene expression and beta-amyloid production, an effect partially reversed by S-adenosylmethionine, a methyl donor favoring DNA methylation [80]. AD has also been associated with miRNAs. MIR-124 is down-regulated in the brain of AD patients [81], and other microRNAs may also be involved. Given the severe and systematic memory impairments associated with AD, these findings strengthen the general role of epigenetics in memory processes.

Similarly, Huntington's disease (HD), though less common and associated with mobility defects in addition to cognitive impairment, also involves epigenetic dysregulation. Like Fragile X syndrome, HD is caused by an abnormal expansion of tri-nucleotide repeats [82]. The resulting extended Huntington (HTT) protein directly binds to CBP and to p300/CBP-associated factor (P/CAF) [83], reducing acetylation of histones 3 and 4 (H3 and H4). MicroRNA dysregulation is also observed in mouse models of HD [84], though it is still not clear if this dysregulation is a cause or consequence of the disease. Again, while only correlative evidence has thus far been established, the striking connection between HD and histone regulation *via* CBP, provides yet another line of support for a role for epigenetics in cognitive functions.

Proteins involved in epigenetic processes have also been linked to several other mental illnesses, including mania and schizophrenia, and may specifically underlie some of the cognitive deficits of these diseases (more details can be found in other chapters in this book). However, like the examples provided above, the association of epigenetics and the diseased brain does not provide information about the precise epigenetic events that serve memory formation. For this reason, investigations using animal models are required to better understand these processes. The following sections describe some of the progress recently achieved.

2.2.2. The Case for DNA Methylation as a "Memory Engram"

The concept that covalent modification of DNA might underlie memory formation [2] is as old as the discovery of DNA methylation itself [1]. In the following sections we describe three basic methodological approaches that have been applied with the aim to better understand the potential role of covalent DNA modifications in memory.

2.2.2.1. Pharmacological Manipulation of DNA Methylation

There are currently no chemical agents that specifically affect proteins directly governing DNA modification. There are however, some non-specific drugs that target enzymes catalyzing the methylation of DNA, and these perturb synaptic plasticity and long-term memory in experimental animals. The DNA methyl transferase (DNMT) inhibitors, 5-aza-deoxycytidine or zebularine, injected in the rat hippocampus immediately after training in fear conditioning prevents contextual fear memory 24 hours later [85]. Similarly, 5-aza-deoxycytidine directly injected in area CA1 of the mouse hippocampus, prevents cocaine-conditioned place preference [86]. However, the DNMT3a inhibitor, RG108, facilitates conditioned place preference when continuously infused in the nucleus accumbens [87], suggesting a role for epigenetic mechanisms in associative memory that may be brain region- and information-specific.

While these pharmacological studies are interesting, they suffer from the lack of specificity of the drugs. DNMT inhibitors are not specific for any DNMT and result in global hypo- or de-methylation of the genome [88]. Such full deregulation of DNA methylation may alter the physiology and functioning of neuronal and glial cells, and interfere with their activity in brain areas important for memory formation [89]. Further, the DNMT inhibitor 5-aza-deoxycytidine can alter the expression profile of genes in organisms that are devoid of DNA methylation such as the common aerobic mold, Aspergillus [90]. Indicating 5-aza-deoxycytidine must also affect processes other than the methylation of DNA. As a result, pharmacological approaches to studying the role of DNA methylation in memory are far from ideal, warranting more specific, targeted experiments using genetic approaches.

2.2.2.2. Genetic Mutations in DNA Methylation Pathways

Thus far, most genetic experiments relevant to the epigenetic machinery have been produced for the purpose of modeling cognitive disease. Rett syndrome results from mutations in MeCP2, a nuclear protein that binds to methylated DNA and the disease is well modeled in mice by genetic inactivation of *Mecp2* [65, 66]. Moreover, the resulting behavioral phenotypes in *Mecp2* nulls can be improved by specific transgenic re-introduction of *Mecp2* to forebrain neurons [91, 92]. As such, mutant mice mimicking all or partial phenotypes for Rett Syndrome, Fragile X Syndrome [93, 94], and Alzheimer's Disease [95] have been generated and together lend strength for a link between careful epigenetic regulation of DNA methylation and the stability of long-term memory.

It is only very recently that mutant animals for a variety of genes in the DNA methylation pathway that are not associated with known disease have been generated and investigated in plasticity and memory paradigms. It is therefore of great interest that along with a global repression of DNA methylation, impairments in long-term synaptic plasticity and long-term memory are observed in double genetic nulls for both mouse *Dnmt1* and *Dnmt3a* [96]. At the same time, because these DNMTs are also important for developmental processes, the double knockout of *Dnmt1* and *Dnmt3a* also reduced neuronal size and led to widespread anomalous gene expression. Considering the resulting neurodevelopmental alterations, it is possible that the cognitive defects derive from the brain abnormalities, and not from a specific effect of perturbing the ability for a neuron to use the covalent modification of DNA as a means of memory formation. It is therefore difficult to judge from this mutant alone, what the effect might be when deregulating DNA methylation during the input-specific stimulation that is usually associated with memory.

2.2.2.3. Direct Measurement of DNA Methylation

If epigenetic processes do take part in the encoding of memory in brain cells, it should be possible to detect epigenetic changes following neural activation known to be associated with memory formation. Further, such epigenetic changes should occur specifically in brain regions that underlie learning and memory. Some of the strongest evidence along this line has come from direct measurements of DNMT activity and DNA methylation.

For example, the level of hippocampal mRNA for *Dnmt3a* and *Dnmt3b,* but not *Dnmt1,* rises by 50-80 % within 30 min after fear conditioning [85], suggesting DNA methylation at some sites may be correspondingly increased. Indeed, in hippocampal area CA1, DNA methylation in the gene coding for a subunit of the memory suppressor, PP1 increases 24 hours after fear conditioning. Importantly, DNA methylation following fear conditioning is not increased at all loci, but also appears to be down-regulated as a function of memory. In particular, the *Reelin* gene, a positive regulator of memory [97], becomes less methylated at its promoter in hippocampus area CA1 following fear conditioning [85]. Moreover, DNA hyper or hypomethylation correlates with performance and is only observed in subjects that formed an association between the context and the foot-shock. Animals given a shock alone but not provided sufficient time to form an associative memory, or animals only exposed to the context and not given a shock, did not demonstrate any change in methylation of the *PP1* or *Reelin* genes, although the subjects likely formed some memory for the shock or the context alone. The data therefore suggest that the methylation events in the promoter regions of *PP1* and *Reelin* are specific for spatial-associative fear memory, and are not recruited for non-spatial-associative fear memory, or non-fearful-associative spatial memory. This specificity of this molecular dissociation is striking.

Changes in DNA methylation on the *Bdnf* gene also occur in neurons of hippocampus area CA1 following both fear memory in a novel context and non-fear memory in a novel context [98]. Yet, only exon IV of *Bdnf* is hypomethylated during formation of fear memory in a novel context, while exons I and VI are hypomethylated during formation of non-fearful memory in a novel context, again demonstrating a strikingly selective regulation of DNA methylation following the formation of specific forms of memory. Such dissociations are the first examples we know to implicate molecular changes that are specifically involved in certain types of memory. These findings underscore that, in addition to the involvement of discrete brain regions in forming specific types of memory, discrete molecular pathways can also be selectively recruited depending on the type of memory being formed. How the brain and individual neurons achieve this type of specificity remains a mystery.

Importantly, DNA hyper and hypomethylation within hippocampus area CA1 seems to be only transient [98]. This is consistent with several studies (for example, see ref. [26]) indicating the hippocampus is critical for the transition of short- to long-term memory, but later dispensable for the storage or the recall of remote events [99]. In the cortex, however, DNA methylation events occur in at least one known memory-related gene, *calcineurin*, and persist for at least 30 days [100], potentially contributing to the storage mechanisms for long-term memory [101]. This transfer of memory is discussed in more detail in later sections and in Box 1.

2.2.3. The Case for Histone Modifications in the Encoding of Memory

Dense chromatin packing is not favorable for efficient gene transcription, and as such, chromatin remodeling can be harnessed by the nucleus as a powerful mechanism to suppress or activate mRNA synthesis. In the mid 1980's, it was demonstrated that the putative nootropic, ethimizol, popular in Russia for its use in pharmacological studies of memory enhancement, affects chromatin structure in the brain [102]. However, an actual role of chromatin remodeling specifically and histone PTMs in chromatin in memory processes has only been revealed in the past decade.

2.2.3.1. Pharmacological Manipulation of Histone PTMs

Like for DNA methylation, several pharmacological agents can be used to manipulate the activity of enzymes that control histone PTMs. Unlike inhibitors of DNMTs however a number of fairly selective drugs targeting histone deacetylases (HDACs) or histone acetyltransferases (HATs) have been identified and are available [103] The principle limitation of HDAC and HAT inhibition comes instead from the fact that these enzymes have many non-histone and non-nuclear acetylation targets, and therefore also interfere with non-nuclear targets that are not closely associated with epigenetics.

When SAHA (suberoylanilide hydroxamic acid), a clinically approved HDAC inhibitor that preferentially targets HDAC2, is administered to adult mice, fear memory both in wild-type animals [104] and in mutant animals modeling Rubinstein-Taybi syndrome through a loss of CBP [105] is improved. The positive effects of SAHA on memory have also been reported in other examples in animals and in the clinic (see review [106]). Importantly, SAHA rescues memory impairment in mice that overexpress *Hdac2*, and does not further enhance memory in knockout mice lacking *Hdac2* [104], supporting an important role for HDAC2 as a negative regulator of memory formation.

Although the pharmacological blockade of HDACs is promising for linking HDAC-dependent processes to the encoding of memory, the approach does not address the potential function of several other histone PTMs including histone phosphorylation, methylation (di and tri) or ubiquitination. Moreover, similar to the application of DNMT inhibitors, only a general effect on the epigenome can be established when applying HDAC inhibitors. Therefore, potential indirect effects on memory formation from globally increasing histone acetylation remain a problem. Just as an example, in addition to their exciting potential as nootropics, HDAC inhibitors have shown promise as cancer therapeutics specifically because of their role in affecting a large number of cytosolic oncogenic processes [107-109]. For this reason, elegant genetic experiments in the mouse are also required when attempting to understand the potential role of histone PTMs in long-term memory formation.

2.2.3.2. Genetic Manipulation of Histone PTMs

Neuron-specific overexpression of *Hdac2* decreases spine density and total synapse number, and alters synaptic plasticity and memory [104], which underscores the importance of HDAC2 in maintaining a neuronal environment amenable to memory formation. Intriguingly, reducing *Hdac2* expression has the opposite effect and induces higher dendritic density, more synapses, facilitated plasticity and enhanced long-term memory. Similar perturbation of *Hdac1* expression does not have any such impact [104], suggesting an important difference in the contribution of HDAC1 and HDAC2 to the structure and function of neurons. One drawback of the knockout experiments, of course, is the potential for developmental abnormalities, since resulting side effects could affect memory formation *via* an epigenetic-independent mechanism. For this reason, the rescue of memory impairments in mice overexpressing HDAC2 with SAFA is important for implicating an acute role for this deacetylase in memory formation. However, whether the effect is truly epigenetic or the result of some non-nuclear or non-histone mechanism still remains to be determined.

It is therefore of great interest that when the memory suppressor PP1 is inhibited selectively in the nucleus of forebrain neurons through inducible transgenic expression of a nucleus-localized inhibitor of PP1, the resulting mice demonstrate enhanced memory in a variety of paradigms [53, 110, 111]. This is of great relevance because the selectivity of the genetic design allows for more precise interpretation of resulting phenotypes, and because PP1 interacts with HDAC1 in cell culture [112], suggesting that it may also do so in adult neurons and could be an important regulator of epigenetic mechanisms critical to memory formation. Consistent with the cell culture findings, following nuclear PP1 inhibition in transgenic mice, PP1 association with neuronal HDAC1 decreases, a change that likely underlies the corresponding increase in acetylation of lysine 14 on H3 (H3K14) and lysine 5 on H4 (H4K5) as well as overall on H2B [110].

In addition to histone acetylation, PP1 also regulates histone phosphorylation in the adult brain [110, 111] and other specific cell types [113]. Inhibition of nuclear PP1 in neurons leads to an increase in phosphorylation of serine 10 on H3 (H3S10) [110], while other phosphorylation sites on H3 are not affected, highlighting a striking degree of residue specificity. Importantly, inhibition of PP1 does not result in any phosphorylation change on synaptic or cytoplasmic targets of PP1, nor on non-histone proteins within the nucleus, such as CREB, MSK1, ERK/MAPK and the chromatin regulators HDAC1 and MeCP2 [110]. As such, the inhibition of nuclear PP1 serves as one of the best lines of evidence for a specific role for epigenetics in memory formation.

Histone trimethylation of H3K36 is also altered in hippocampal neurons following inhibition of nuclear PP1, likely as a result of a novel association discovered between PP1 and the histone demethylase, JMJD2A (jumonji domain-containing protein 2A) [110]. Finally, inhibition of nuclear PP1 in the forebrain affects histone PTMs and facilitates synaptic plasticity in the amygdala; molecular and cellular changes that occur concurrently with the phenotype of enhanced fear memory [111]. Together, these findings highlight an important role for multiple epigenetic marks on protein histones in memory formation.

Yet, as seems to be the case for DNA methylation events, histone modifications underlying memory should, at least in theory, demonstrate loci specificity. Already some progress has been made in this direction in the context of PP1 by comparing the expression profile of key memory genes with and without nuclear inhibition of PP1. For example, the promoter region of *Creb* carries histones with increased phosphorylation, acetylation and trimethylation on the same residues modified by PP1, and the transcription of *Creb* is increased as a result of inhibition of nuclear PP1 [110, 114]. In contrast, the genes such as NFκB (nuclear factor-κB) have less histone PTMs on their promoters, and are expressed at a lower level following nuclear PP1 inhibition. The phenomenon of bidirectional control over gene transcription by PP1 appears to be a genome-wide effect, since high-throughput microarray analyses of hippocampus extracts reveal a comparable number of genes either up- or down-regulated following selective inhibition of the PP1 protein in neuron nuclei.

2.2.3.3. Direct Measurement of Histone PTMs

If histone PTMs and chromatin remodeling are part of the process of memory formation, these events should be measurable during or immediately after events that are known to lead to memory. Consistent with this idea, pulse application of serotonin to the *Aplysia* sensory neuron that results in long-term synaptic facilitation and mimics learning [115], also increases acetylation of both H4K8 and H3K14 within the CAAT box enhancer binding protein (C/EBP) promoter [116]. Acetylation of these histones at the C/EBP promoter is also associated with increased transcription of the C/EBP gene, suggesting that chromatin remodeling is a mechanism by which neurons mediate long-term facilitation. Interestingly, transcription of C/EBP and acetylation of H3 and H4 is transient, the time-dependence of which correlates well with the presence of CREB1 and CBP at the promoter of C/EBP. In turn, deacetylation of H3 and H4 correlates in time with the recruitment of CREB2 and HDAC5 to the promoter region of C/EBP. Importantly, the exact reverse effects are observed when, instead of serotonin, the inhibitory transmitter FMRFamide that induces long-term depression is applied to sensory neurons, demonstrating bidirectional control of C/EBP gene transcription through histone acetylation/deacetylation [116].

In mammals, just as in *Aplysia*, long-term synaptic changes in efficacy are believed to underlie the process of memory formation. Therefore, if epigenetic events contribute to synaptic efficacy, specific alterations in the profile of PTMs of histones might occur following training in learning and memory paradigms. In support of this, H3S10 phosphorylation is increased following fear conditioning [117]. Moreover, at the promoter site for CREB, phosphorylation of H3S10, acetylation of H3K14, and trimethylation of H3K36 increases following training on an object recognition task [110]. In contrast, acetylation of H3K9 and H3K14 decreases at the same locus following training. If these particular histone PTMs contribute to the encoding of long-term memory, mutant mice with enhanced learning and memory might also shown enhanced changes in histone PTMs at the CREB promoter, as a means to biochemically elevate CREB transcription. Indeed, nuclear inhibition of PP1, which improves memory, also increases these modifications on histones at the CREB promoter [110]. Together, these findings point to a critical role for histone PTMs in memory formation.

2.2.4. The Case for microRNAs as Mediators of Synaptic Memory

Perhaps the most appealing argument for microRNAs playing a critical role in memory formation is the ability of microRNAs to locally control protein synthesis [6, 118]. In this way, microRNAs may serve as one of several synaptic tags and provide for the synapse-specificity that is considered to be integral to memory. For recent reviews of the synaptic-specificity hypothesis and the likely role for microRNAs in this process, we refer the reader to references [119, 120]. Of course, microRNAs not only play a role in dendrites, but are also present in the developing axons of neurons [121, 122], where functional RISCs (RNA-induced silencing complexes) can also be found [123].

2.2.4.1. Pharmacological Manipulation of microRNAs

Pharmacological antagonism of specific microRNAs is fairly straightforward when compared to the pharmacological antagonism of proteins. Unlike proteins, the anti-sense strands of microRNAs, or "antagomirs", are able to inhibit the function of selected microRNAs [124]. These inhibitors of microRNAs also benefit from having few side effects, although multiple targets can be affected since individual microRNA often target several transcripts (for example, see [125]). A variety of modifications to the nucleic acid backbone, or to nucleic acids themselves, have proven useful for both extending the half-life and increasing the efficacy of microRNA antagonists (for review see ref. [126]).

The antagomir approach has been successfully applied to study the role of microRNAs in neuronal morphology, plasticity and animal behavior of invertebrates as well as mammals. An antisense 2'-O-methyl-oligoribonucleotide antagomir against mIR-12 in *Aplysia*, for example, enhances long-term facilitation and increases CREB translation [127], underscoring the importance of endogenous mIR-12 as a suppressor of CREB translation *in vivo*. An antagomir against the CREB-controlled microRNA, miR-132, on the other hand, attenuates neurite outgrowth in rat cortical neuron cultures [118]. Indeed, in many of the investigations carried out on microRNAs, antagomir approaches have been applied to target specific transcripts.

General pharmacological targeting of microRNA pathways has not yet been applied owing to an absence of blockers against the key enzymes, including Drosha or Dicer. Instead, to address broad questions regarding the overall importance of microRNAs to the processes of plasticity and memory, some experimenters have taken a genetic approach.

2.2.4.2. Genetic Manipulation of microRNAs

Few genetic knockout studies have been carried out on the specific genes encoding microRNAs. This is in part because a role for microRNAs in brain plasticity is still a relatively new concept, and in part because microRNAs are often encoded in the introns of other genes, and therefore difficult to target specifically. In addition to these individual microRNA-selective mutants, proteins involved in microRNA processing have also been targeted [128]. Deletion of *Dicer1* in the adult murine forebrain is associated with an enhancement in hippocampal-dependent learning and elevated expression of memory-related genes such as *Bdnf* and *Psd95* [128]. However, LTP in area CA1 of the hippocampus is unchanged in the absence of *Dicer1*, an observation that may indicate that facilitation of plasticity in other hippocampal subregions underlie the observed memory enhancements. Enhancement in spatial learning is also found, for example, when synaptic plasticity is facilitated in the dentate gyrus but unchanged in area CA1, as is true following induced overexpression of *Ncs1* in the adult mouse dentate gyrus [15].

Although not part of the microRNA generating machinery, the deacetylase SIRT1 regulates the expression of several microRNAs. However, unlike Dicer1, SIRT1 has direct control over microRNA transcription through a Yin Yang 1 (YY1) transcription factor repressor complex [129]. Loss-of-function SIRT1 mutant mice demonstrate impaired hippocampal-dependent learning, fewer dendritic spines in

CA1 pyramidal neurons, and a lack of LTP in CA1 [129]. Of the several microRNAs controlled by SIRT1, is miR-134, an important regulator of neural differentiation [130] and spine development through the protein kinase Limk1 and BDNF [6]. Direct lentiviral delivery of miR-134 to the hippocampus of mice impairs LTP and fear conditioning, mimicking the SIRT1 loss-of-function phenotype. Importantly, blockade of miR-134 in the loss-of-function animals rescues both the long-term synaptic plasticity and fear memory impairments [129], suggesting that although genetic mutation of SIRT1 alters the expression of many microRNA, the change in expression of miR-134 alone is both sufficient to induce, as well as rescue, similar phenotypes. Most intriguingly, since miR-134 acts to regulate BDNF expression [6], and local BDNF expression at synapses may be critical to the generation of synaptic specificity [131], locally isolated miR-134 itself could also be a key component of the synapse-specific plasticity events that are believed to underlie memory [132, 133] (see Fig. **2**).

Overexpression and repression of two microRNAs that interact with fragile X mental retardation protein, miR-125b and miR-132, affects dendritic spine morphology [75]. Interestingly, the NMDA receptor subunit NR2A appears to be a direct target of miR-125b, since antagonism and overexpression of miR-125b can regulate both *Nr2a* expression levels, as well as NMDA receptor currents [75].

At the same time, genetic forebrain overexpression of miR-132 in mice impairs object recognition memory, while increasing spine density in hippocampal subregion CA1 [69], demonstrating that individual microRNA can have profound effects on both cognition and neuronal morphology. These findings help partially explain phenotypes in *Dicer* null mice, in which miR-132 expression is suppressed [128]. Interestingly, the DNA methylation protein, MeCP2 seems to be a target for miR-132 since expression of MeCP2 is decreased in miR-132 overexpressing mice [69], a finding that underscores a complex interconnectivity orchestrated between various epigenetic mechanisms. The interplay between distinct forms of epigenetics is a re-occurring theme that appears to be critical for memory formation.

2.2.4.3. Direct Measurement of microRNAs

The machinery required for microRNAs to exert their effect on mRNA transcripts is present not only in neuron cell bodies, where most translation occurs, but also in the axons [121, 122] and dendrites [134] of neurons, suggesting that microRNAs locally control the transcription of proteins important for synaptic communication.

Two hours following induction of LTP in the dentate gyrus of rats, a brain region critical to spontaneous exploration of novel environments and spatial learning [15], miR-132 and miR-212 are expressed at 50 times their pre-induction levels [135]. Serotonin application to the sensory neurons of *Aplysia* that leads to long-term facilitation reduces the expression of miR-124 [127]. Armitage, a key component of the microRNA silencing complex is localized to synapses in *Drosophila* neurons, and is degraded following neural activity or learning, an effect that governs the expression of CaMKII [136]. Very likely, these findings represent only a small part of the major and the many roles for microRNAs in plasticity and memory, roles that are just now beginning to be revealed.

2.3. MODELS FOR EPIGENETIC REGULATION OF MEMORY

As demonstrated above, epigenetic mechanisms clearly play a fundamental role in learning and memory given that: 1) cognitive impairments in the diseased are often associated with compromised epigenetic machinery and processes; 2) drugs that interfere with epigenetic pathways can bidirectionally affect memory; 3) genetic mutations in epigenetic-relevant genes can also impair or improve memory in animals; and 4) after learning, reproducible epigenetic changes are found to occur in the animal brain, and are sometimes localized to synaptic regions.

Using this conceptual basis, we can now again approach the question formulated by Griffith and Mahler in their 1969 hypothesis [2], but this time instead of asking *if* epigenetics play a role in memory, we ask *how*. How exactly do epigenetic mechanisms control learning and memory? Are some forms of memory, or specific brain regions, more dependent on epigenetic regulation? What might be the signaling pathways underlying these epigenetic changes? Is the epigenetic regulatory machinery a suitable target for pharmaceuticals? Can we use epigenetics to reverse cognitive defects associated with mental illness? Could general regulators of epigenetic processes serve as cognitive enhancers in non-diseased individuals?

It is now increasingly apparent that the epigenetic regulation of neuronal structures and functions, of brain plasticity and of processes leading to memory formation, are probably universally orchestrated by the intertwining of covalent DNA tagging, histone posttranslational modification, chromatin remodeling, and microRNAs. Drugs that target the DNA methylation machinery, for example, indirectly affect the profile of histone PTMs. This is the case for FMR1 gene activation by the DNMT inhibitor 5-aza-deoxycytidine, which also increases dimethylation and acetylation of H3 at the FMR1 gene loci [137]. 5-aza-deoxycytidine also increases overall H4 acetylation, while decreasing overall H3K9 dimethylation [79]. Another striking example involves the link between microRNAs and DNA methylation, where expression of the brain specific microRNA, miR-184 is controlled by MeCP2, a methyl DNA binding protein that can act as an activator or repressor of gene expression [138]. Binding of MeCP2 to the promoter of miR-184 decreases following neuron depolarization, which leads to miR-184 synthesis, revealing another means through which DNA methylation contributes to microRNA expression. These examples are far more likely to be the rule, rather than the exception, as neurons can recruit multiple mechanisms for the fine-tuned establishment and maintenance of memory.

Enzymes of the chromatin machinery therefore, such as PP1, likely have a dual role in the control of gene expression. Future studies based on mouse models in which specific components of the machinery are manipulated selectively in the nucleus and in restricted cell populations, for instance hippocampal or cortical neurons, will be instrumental in further delineating the combined role of epigenetics in memory formation. Highly selective manipulations will best help understand the intimate mechanisms of the epigenetic machinery underlying memory, since existing knockout, knock-down, overexpression or pharmacological studies are confounded by the fact that non-epigenetic targets are also affected.

Additional forms of histone modifications, such as O-linked N-acetylglycosylation (O-GlcNAc) [139], could also be involved in memory processes, as could several other types of modifications known to occur on histones in the brain [140]. The investigation of these lesser-studied histone PTMs on gene transcription will be an area of intense focus in the future.

Using the data currently available, we have generated an evolving model for the epigenetic regulation of memory centering on the activation of NMDA receptors and the resulting expression of CREB (Fig. **2**).

Box1 | Epigenetic Support of a Memory Engram

As noted by Ebbinghaus over a century ago, following initial encoding (stage 1), memory can return to consciousness either on demand or spontaneously, and frequently with high fidelity. One possible explanation for "memory-readiness" is that memory may be stored in both a biochemical and electrical form.

In other words, memory might exist as a biochemically-supported electrical engram or "reverberation" (stage 2) of the initial experience. Of particular relevance to this chapter, some of the major biochemical events underlying the long-term stability of this engram could be epigenetic in nature.

In order to achieve a stable electrical circuit, neurons of the circuit must fire asynchronously, since asynchronous firing allows the activation of one neuron to trigger activation of the next neuron, and eventually complete (and re-initiate) the circuit. Yet, some brain wave activity, including the slow wave propagation of depressive activity that occurs during slow-wave sleep (stage 3), is incompatible with asynchronous neuronal firing. Slow-wave sleep therefore poses a problem for memory being stored as an active electrical engram, since the accompanying slow wave depression would be predicted to stop the engram (thereby erasing the memory). Epigenetic events however, might not be disrupted by slow-wave sleep, and could therefore help establish synaptic weights so that once asynchronous activity is again viable, the priming of a subset of neurons can re-activate the engram. Thus, epigenetics might be critical to returning a memory engram to an active state that is immediately accessible to conscious processing (stage 4).

A model that includes the active storage of a memory engram allows for re-molding of the neuronal network without loss of memory. Thus over time, the storage of memory could become increasingly efficient in terms of the number of neurons and biochemical events required to stabilize the engram (stages 4-6). Additionally and/or alternatively, an active memory engram might be free to transfer to new regions of the brain where novel sets of epigenetic events might stabilize an evolving engram.

The proposed model of memory therefore does not demand the indefinite persistence of any individual neuron, synapse or epigenetic event. Thus, biochemical redundancy within the system is also possible, and several epigenetic events might be employed for stabilizing a single memory engram.

Legend

 Active neuron, asynchronous network firing

 Inactive neuron, not part of activity network

 Neuron active during slow-wave spreading

→ Active synaptic communication

→ Slow-wave synaptic spreading

Epigenetic events, including DNA methylation, histone post-translational modifications, and the synthesis or inhibition of microRNAs

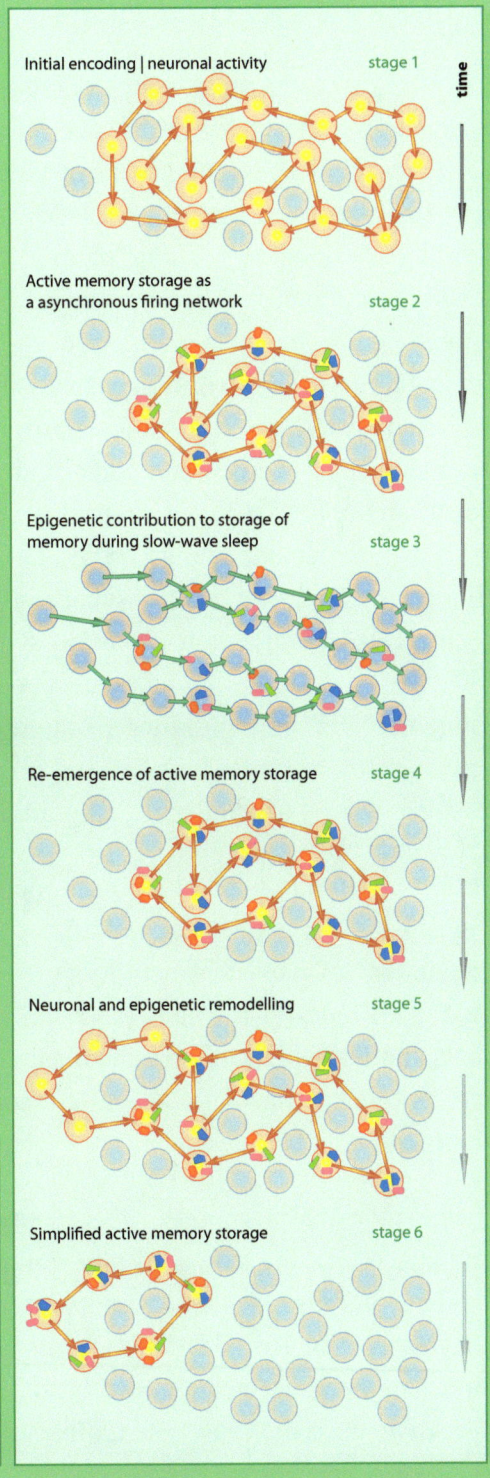

Initial encoding | neuronal activity   stage 1

time

Active memory storage as a asynchronous firing network   stage 2

Epigenetic contribution to storage of memory during slow-wave sleep   stage 3

Re-emergence of active memory storage   stage 4

Neuronal and epigenetic remodelling   stage 5

Simplified active memory storage   stage 6

2.4. UNRESOLVED QUESTIONS

One obvious conceptual issue related to the idea of an enduring individual epigenetic change serving as a specific memory trace, is the problem of memory specificity. Currently, one prevalent view in neuroscience is that synapses are the most likely storage site for memory traces, or at least that synapse-specific plasticity is critical to accurate memory formation, maintenance and recall [119]. As such, an individual synapse could code for a specific feature, or "bit" of a memory. This theory is supported by mathematical models that consider the estimated 100 to 200 trillion synapses in the human neocortex provide sufficient individual bits to make up the entire wealth of memory in any given human. However, while neurons can contain around 7,000 synapses, they have only one nucleus and only two copies of most genes. If each specific feature of a memory is stored as a molecular change on the DNA itself, each could be expected to exert influence over all of the cell's synapses, unless the cell has some way of coupling specific DNA methylation events to specific synapses. In the absence of such a molecular connection, the storage of memory in DNA itself does not match the requirement for multiple sites of storage per neuron, and essentially dedicates each neuron to a single bit of stored information, reducing the overall number of storable bits by 4 or 5 orders of magnitude.

Another possibility is that long-term memory traces may not be stored exclusively in synapses or *via* covalent modification of the DNA, but instead, may be the embodiment of persistent activity, such as is often theorized to be the case for working memory [141]. It is possible that DNA modifications, other epigenetic events and non-epigenetic biochemical changes in the nucleus or at synapses only serve as transient mediators of an electrical memory engram, as explained below and described in Box 1.

To illustrate this possibility, it is helpful to consider the potential for artificial intelligence. At the dawn of the computer revolution, it was calculated that encoding 30 bits of memory per second continuously for 100 years requires enough space for 10^{11} (100 billion) bits [142], which is approximately equal to the number of neurons in the entire brain. And although 100 billion seems like an impressive number, it is potentially still insufficient to encode the richness of human experience. 100 billion bytes (100 GB), for example, represent less than a half-day of high definition video. As such, it might not be reasonable to assume that a single neuron, or even a single synapse, represents any particular bit of memory in the human brain.

To use another analogy, synaptic changes and DNA modifications might be better compared to the words of a book. In this example, the ideas of the book (not the words) are what is typically viewed as memory. As such, the precise words selected are not critical, since the same meaning can often be expressed through the combination of a variety of different words. Similarly, the precise chemical changes that occur in the brain may not correspond directly to any bit of memory, but instead combine to maintain persistent and asynchronous neuron activity. In this way, the physical basis of memory in the brain could be non-static and multiply redundant, which is consistent with a variety of fundamental findings in memory research.

By its very design, the brain's fundamental difference from all other organs of the body is its exceptional ability to use electrical communication for elaborate, dynamic and flexible signaling. The nervous system, which supports functions such as cognition, self-awareness, and love, may have this ability not because neurons do not divide, but instead because it can propagate electrical activity. The observation that approximate 1% of the brain's 100 billion neurons engaged in active firing at any given instant during wakefulness and sleep [143] could suggest that neuronal activity is occurring beyond the mere need for maintaining bodily functions or thinking. The continual active firing of 1 billion neurons might instead represent memory.

This enduring propagation of neuronal activity theory for memory is also consistent with the immediacy with which memories can be returned to consciousness, as observed by Ebbinghaus [7]. If a bit of information were stored in DNA, on the other hand, is it difficult to imagine how exactly this bit of information could suddenly burst into consciousness in concert with millions of other bits, as is experienced daily in humans. Yet, epigenetic mechanisms and synaptic restructuring events could be critical to the re-establishment of electrical memory engrams after sleep or injury, since although the total amount of neuronal activity does not change drastically between sleep and wake states, the characteristics of neuronal activity do change [143], and therefore an electrical memory engram might be lost in the process. In this way, memory might be stored as both a chemical change and an electrical propagation, depending on the overall brain state. This theory is consistent with the familiar feeling of being unable to immediately access memories when waking from a deep sleep.

The theory is also consistent with the observation that memory again becomes dependent on protein synthesis following re-activation [144]. It is therefore possible that reconsolidation also involves epigenetic events, a finding that might emphasize the importance of persistent neuronal activity as a long-term storage mechanism for memory.

CONCLUSIONS

Epigenetic regulation of gene transcription and translation, through direct DNA modification, histone/chromatin remodeling, and microRNAs, is emerging as a central process in the establishment and maintenance of memory. This is especially owing to the enduring nature of many epigenetic processes. The ability of microRNAs to act locally at synapses is a particularly intriguing phenomenon and will be the focus of intense research in the coming years. Together, the emergence of epigenetic research in the neurosciences is revolutionizing how we view the brain.

REFERENCES

[1]   Barondes SH, Cohen HD. Puromycin effect on successive phases of memory storage. Science 1966; 151: 594-5.
[2]   Griffith JS, Mahler HR. DNA ticketing theory of memory. Nature 1969; 223: 580-2.
[3]   Crick F. Memory and molecular turnover. Nature 1984; 312: 101.
[4]   Holliday R. Is there an epigenetic component in long-term memory? J Theor Biol 1999; 200: 339-41.
[5]   Bruce D. Fifty years since Lashley's In search of the Engram: refutations and conjectures. J Hist Neurosci 2001; 10: 308-18.
[6]   Schratt GM, Tuebing F, Nigh EA, Kane CG, Sabatini ME, Kiebler M, *et al.* A brain-specific microRNA regulates dendritic spine development. Nature 2006; 439: 283-9.
[7]   Ebbinghaus H. Ueder das Gedachtniss, experimentelle Untersuchungen: Leipzig, Verlag Von Duncken & Hemblot; 1885.
[8]   James W. The Principles of Psychology Boston: Harvard University Press; 1890.
[9]   Milner B, Penfield W. The effect of hippocampal lesions on recent memory. Trans Am Neurol Assoc 1955(80th Meeting): 42-8.

[10]   Penfield W, Milner B. Memory deficit produced by bilateral lesions in the hippocampal zone. AMA Arch Neurol Psychiatry 1958; 79: 475-97.

[11]   Scoville WB, Milner B. Loss of recent memory after bilateral hippocampal lesions. J Neurol Neurosurg Psychiatry 1957; 20: 11-21.

[12]   Alvarez P, Zola-Morgan S, Squire LR. Damage limited to the hippocampal region produces long-lasting memory impairment in monkeys. J Neurosci 1995; 15: 3796-807.

[13]   Dzidzishvili NN, Ungiadze AA, Davituliani D. [The effect of dorsal and ventral hippocampal lesions on short-term memory in cats]. Zh Vyssh Nerv Deiat Im I P Pavlova 1975; 25: 70-7.

[14]   Ross RT, Orr WB, Holland PC, Berger TW. Hippocampectomy disrupts acquisition and retention of learned conditional responding. Behav Neurosci 1984; 98: 211-25.

[15]   Saab BJ, Georgiou J, Nath A, Lee FJ, Wang M, Michalon A, *et al.* NCS-1 in the dentate gyrus promotes exploration, synaptic plasticity, and rapid acquisition of spatial memory. Neuron 2009; 63: 643-56.

[16]   Zola-Morgan S, Squire LR. Memory impairment in monkeys following lesions limited to the hippocampus. Behav Neurosci 1986; 100: 155-60.

[17]   Flexner LB, Flexner JB, Roberts RB, Delahaba G. Loss of Recent Memory in Mice as Related to Regional Inhibition of Cerebral Protein Synthesis. Proc Natl Acad Sci U S A 1964; 52: 1165-9.

[18]   Krug M, Lossner B, Ott T. Anisomycin blocks the late phase of long-term potentiation in the dentate gyrus of freely moving rats. Brain Res Bull 1984; 13: 39-42.

[19]   Mizumori SJ, Channon V, Rosenzweig MR, Bennett EL. Anisomycin impairs long-term working memory in a delayed alternation task. Behav Neural Biol 1987; 47: 1-6.

[20]   Stanton PK, Sarvey JM. Blockade of long-term potentiation in rat hippocampal CA1 region by inhibitors of protein synthesis. J Neurosci 1984; 4: 3080-8.

[21]   Hebb DO. The organization of behavior; a neuropsychological theory. New York,: Wiley; 1949.

[22]   Bliss TV, Gardner-Medwin AR. Long-lasting potentiation of synaptic transmission in the dentate area of the unanaestetized rabbit following stimulation of the perforant path. J Physiol 1973; 232: 357-74.

[23]   Bliss TV, Lomo T. Long-lasting potentiation of synaptic transmission in the dentate area of the anaesthetized rabbit following stimulation of the perforant path. J Physiol 1973; 232: 331-56.

[24]   Nguyen PV, Abel T, Kandel ER, Bourtchouladze R. Strain-dependent differences in LTP and hippocampus-dependent memory in inbred mice. Learn Mem 2000; 7: 170-9.

[25]   Malleret G, Haditsch U, Genoux D, Jones MW, Bliss TV, Vanhoose AM, *et al.* Inducible and reversible enhancement of learning, memory, and long-term potentiation by genetic inhibition of calcineurin. Cell 2001; 104: 675-86.

[26]   Mansuy IM, Mayford M, Jacob B, Kandel ER, Bach ME. Restricted and regulated overexpression reveals calcineurin as a key component in the transition from short-term to long-term memory. Cell 1998; 92: 39-49.

[27]   Lehrer J. Neuroscience: Small, furry.and smart. Nature 2009; 461: 862-4.

[28]   Lee HK, Takamiya K, Han JS, Man H, Kim CH, Rumbaugh G, *et al.* Phosphorylation of the AMPA receptor GluR1 subunit is required for synaptic plasticity and retention of spatial memory. Cell 2003; 112: 631-43.

[29]   Whitlock JR, Heynen AJ, Shuler MG, Bear MF. Learning induces long-term potentiation in the hippocampus. Science 2006; 313: 1093-7.

[30]   Amaral DG, Witter MP. The three-dimensional organization of the hippocampal formation: a review of anatomical data. Neuroscience 1989; 31: 571-91.

[31]   Andersen P, Holmqvist B, Voorhoeve PE. Excitatory synapses on hippocampal apical dendrites activated by entorhinal stimulation. Acta Physiol Scand 1966; 66: 461-72.

[32]   Nong Y, Huang YQ, Ju W, Kalia LV, Ahmadian G, Wang YT, *et al.* Glycine binding primes NMDA receptor internalization. Nature 2003; 422: 302-7.

[33]   Harris EW, Ganong AH, Cotman CW. Long-term potentiation in the hippocampus involves activation of N-methyl-D-aspartate receptors. Brain Res 1984; 323: 132-7.

[34]   Mayer ML, Westbrook GL, Guthrie PB. Voltage-dependent block by Mg2+ of NMDA responses in spinal cord neurones. Nature 1984; 309: 261-3.

[35]   Sarvey JM, Burgard EC, Decker G. Long-term potentiation: studies in the hippocampal slice. J Neurosci Methods 1989; 28: 109-24.

[36]   Abraham WC, Mason SE. Effects of the NMDA receptor/channel antagonists CPP and MK801 on hippocampal field potentials and long-term potentiation in anesthetized rats. Brain Res 1988; 462: 40-6.

[37]   Danysz W, Wroblewski JT, Costa E. Learning impairment in rats by N-methyl-D-aspartate receptor antagonists. Neuropharmacology 1988; 27: 653-6.

[38]   Benvenga MJ, Spaulding TC. Amnesic effect of the novel anticonvulsant MK-801. Pharmacol Biochem Behav 1988; 30: 205-7.

[39]   Worley PF, Bhat RV, Baraban JM, Erickson CA, McNaughton BL, Barnes CA. Thresholds for synaptic activation of transcription factors in hippocampus: correlation with long-term enhancement. J Neurosci 1993; 13: 4776-86.

[40]   Kasahara J, Fukunaga K, Miyamoto E. Activation of calcium/calmodulin-dependent protein kinase IV in long term potentiation in the rat hippocampal CA1 region. J Biol Chem 2001; 276: 24044-50.

[41]   Dash PK, Hochner B, Kandel ER. Injection of the cAMP-responsive element into the nucleus of Aplysia sensory neurons blocks long-term facilitation. Nature 1990; 345: 718-21.

[42]   Bourtchuladze R, Frenguelli B, Blendy J, Cioffi D, Schutz G, Silva AJ. Deficient long-term memory in mice with a targeted mutation of the cAMP-responsive element-binding protein. Cell 1994; 79: 59-68.

[43]   Ying SW, Futter M, Rosenblum K, Webber MJ, Hunt SP, Bliss TV, *et al.* Brain-derived neurotrophic factor induces long-term potentiation in intact adult hippocampus: requirement for ERK activation coupled to CREB and upregulation of Arc synthesis. J Neurosci 2002; 22: 1532-40.

[44]   Impey S, Obrietan K, Wong ST, Poser S, Yano S, Wayman G, *et al.* Cross talk between ERK and PKA is required for Ca2+ stimulation of CREB-dependent transcription and ERK nuclear translocation. Neuron 1998; 21: 869-83.

[45]   Genoux D, Haditsch U, Knobloch M, Michalon A, Storm D, Mansuy IM. Protein phosphatase 1 is a molecular constraint on learning and memory. Nature 2002; 418: 970-5.

[46]   Phillips AG, LePiane FG. Reinforcing effects of morphine microinjection into the ventral tegmental area. Pharmacol Biochem Behav 1980; 12: 965-8.

[47]   Zvartau EE, Kovalenko VS. [Secondary-reinforcing effects of opiate agonists in the mouse]. Zh Vyssh Nerv Deiat Im I P Pavlova 1986; 36: 1069-76.

[48]   Baron A. Suppression of Exploratory Behavior by Aversive Stimulation. J Comp Physiol Psychol 1964; 57: 299-301.

[49]   Morris R. Developments of a water-maze procedure for studying spatial learning in the rat. J Neurosci Methods 1984; 11: 47-60.

[50] Saab BJ, Saab AM, Roder JC. Statistical and theoretical considerations for the platform relocation water maze. J Neurosci Methods 2011; 198: 44-52.

[51] Berlyne DE. Novelty and curiosity as determinants of exploratory behaviour. Br J Psychol 1950; 41: 68-80.

[52] Becker JT, Olton DS, Anderson CA, Breitinger ER. Cognitive mapping in rats: the role of the hippocampal and frontal system in retention and reversal. Behav Brain Res 1981; 3: 1-22.

[53] Graff J, Mansuy IM. Epigenetic codes in cognition and behaviour. Behav Brain Res 2008; 192: 70-87.

[54] Saab BJ, Roder JC. Normalizing Endophenotypes of Schizophrenia: The Dip and Draw Hypothesis. Hypothesis 2007; 5: 23-9.

[55] Petrij F, Giles RH, Dauwerse HG, Saris JJ, Hennekam RC, Masuno M, *et al.* Rubinstein-Taybi syndrome caused by mutations in the transcriptional co-activator CBP. Nature 1995; 376: 348-51.

[56] Alberini CM. Transcription factors in long-term memory and synaptic plasticity. Physiol Rev 2009; 89: 121-45.

[57] Bannister AJ, Kouzarides T. The CBP co-activator is a histone acetyltransferase. Nature 1996; 384: 641-3.

[58] Oike Y, Hata A, Mamiya T, Kaname T, Noda Y, Suzuki M, *et al.* Truncated CBP protein leads to classical Rubinstein-Taybi syndrome phenotypes in mice: implications for a dominant-negative mechanism. Hum Mol Genet 1999; 8: 387-96.

[59] Korzus E, Rosenfeld MG, Mayford M. CBP histone acetyltransferase activity is a critical component of memory consolidation. Neuron 2004; 42: 961-72.

[60] Roelfsema JH, White SJ, Ariyurek Y, Bartholdi D, Niedrist D, Papadia F, *et al.* Genetic heterogeneity in Rubinstein-Taybi syndrome: mutations in both the CBP and EP300 genes cause disease. Am J Hum Genet 2005; 76: 572-80.

[61] Kalkhoven E, Roelfsema JH, Teunissen H, den Boer A, Ariyurek Y, Zantema A, *et al.* Loss of CBP acetyltransferase activity by PHD finger mutations in Rubinstein-Taybi syndrome. Hum Mol Genet 2003; 12: 441-50.

[62] Murata T, Kurokawa R, Krones A, Tatsumi K, Ishii M, Taki T, *et al.* Defect of histone acetyltransferase activity of the nuclear transcriptional coactivator CBP in Rubinstein-Taybi syndrome. Hum Mol Genet 2001; 10: 1071-6.

[63] Percy AK. Rett syndrome: recent research progress. J Child Neurol 2008; 23: 543-9.

[64] Amir RE, Van den Veyver IB, Wan M, Tran CQ, Francke U, Zoghbi HY. Rett syndrome is caused by mutations in X-linked MECP2, encoding methyl-CpG-binding protein 2. Nat Genet 1999; 23: 185-8.

[65] Chen RZ, Akbarian S, Tudor M, Jaenisch R. Deficiency of methyl-CpG binding protein-2 in CNS neurons results in a Rett-like phenotype in mice. Nat Genet 2001; 27: 327-31.

[66] Guy J, Hendrich B, Holmes M, Martin JE, Bird A. A mouse Mecp2-null mutation causes neurological symptoms that mimic Rett syndrome. Nat Genet 2001; 27: 322-6.

[67] Adkins NL, Georgel PT. MeCP2: structure and function. Biochem Cell Biol 2011; 89: 1-11.

[68] Dragich J, Houwink-Manville I, Schanen C. Rett syndrome: a surprising result of mutation in MECP2. Hum Mol Genet 2000; 9: 2365-75.

[69] Hansen KF, Sakamoto K, Wayman GA, Impey S, Obrietan K. Transgenic miR132 alters neuronal spine density and impairs novel object recognition memory. PLoS One 2010; 5: e15497.

[70]   Wu H, Tao J, Chen PJ, Shahab A, Ge W, Hart RP, *et al.* Genome-wide analysis reveals methyl-CpG-binding protein 2-dependent regulation of microRNAs in a mouse model of Rett syndrome. Proc Natl Acad Sci U S A 2010; 107: 18161-6.

[71]   Urdinguio RG, Fernandez AF, Lopez-Nieva P, Rossi S, Huertas D, Kulis M, *et al.* Disrupted microRNA expression caused by Mecp2 loss in a mouse model of Rett syndrome. Epigenetics 2010; 5: 656-63.

[72]   Ashley CT, Sutcliffe JS, Kunst CB, Leiner HA, Eichler EE, Nelson DL, *et al.* Human and murine FMR-1: alternative splicing and translational initiation downstream of the CGG-repeat. Nat Genet 1993; 4: 244-51.

[73]   Gu Y, Shen Y, Gibbs RA, Nelson DL. Identification of FMR2, a novel gene associated with the FRAXE CCG repeat and CpG island. Nat Genet 1996; 13: 109-13.

[74]   Gecz J, Gedeon AK, Sutherland GR, Mulley JC. Identification of the gene FMR2, associated with FRAXE mental retardation. Nat Genet 1996; 13: 105-8.

[75]   Edbauer D, Neilson JR, Foster KA, Wang CF, Seeburg DP, Batterton MN, *et al.* Regulation of synaptic structure and function by FMRP-associated microRNAs miR-125b and miR-132. Neuron 2010; 65: 373-84.

[76]   Cheever A, Blackwell E, Ceman S. Fragile X protein family member FXR1P is regulated by microRNAs. RNA 2010; 16: 1530-9.

[77]   Cheever A, Ceman S. Phosphorylation of FMRP inhibits association with Dicer. RNA 2009; 15: 362-6.

[78]   Ballard C, Gauthier S, Corbett A, Brayne C, Aarsland D, Jones E. Alzheimer's disease. Lancet 2011; 377: 1019-31.

[79]   Marambaud P, Wen PH, Dutt A, Shioi J, Takashima A, Siman R, *et al.* A CBP binding transcriptional repressor produced by the PS1/epsilon-cleavage of N-cadherin is inhibited by PS1 FAD mutations. Cell 2003; 114: 635-45.

[80]   Scarpa S, Fuso A, D'Anselmi F, Cavallaro RA. Presenilin 1 gene silencing by S-adenosylmethionine: a treatment for Alzheimer disease? FEBS Lett 2003; 541: 145-8.

[81]   Smith P, Al Hashimi A, Girard J, Delay C, Hebert SS. *In vivo* regulation of amyloid precursor protein neuronal splicing by microRNAs. J Neurochem 2011; 116: 240-7.

[82]   Bates GP. History of genetic disease: the molecular genetics of Huntington disease - a history. Nat Rev Genet 2005; 6: 766-73.

[83]   Steffan JS, Bodai L, Pallos J, Poelman M, McCampbell A, Apostol BL, *et al.* Histone deacetylase inhibitors arrest polyglutamine-dependent neurodegeneration in Drosophila. Nature 2001; 413: 739-43.

[84]   Lee ST, Chu K, Im WS, Yoon HJ, Im JY, Park JE, *et al.* Altered microRNA regulation in Huntington's disease models. Exp Neurol 2011; 227: 172-9.

[85]   Miller CA, Sweatt JD. Covalent modification of DNA regulates memory formation. Neuron 2007; 53: 857-69.

[86]   Han J, Li Y, Wang D, Wei C, Yang X, Sui N. Effect of 5-aza-2-deoxycytidine microinjecting into hippocampus and prelimbic cortex on acquisition and retrieval of cocaine-induced place preference in C57BL/6 mice. Eur J Pharmacol 2010; 642: 93-8.

[87]   LaPlant Q, Vialou V, Covington HE, 3rd, Dumitriu D, Feng J, Warren BL, *et al.* Dnmt3a regulates emotional behavior and spine plasticity in the nucleus accumbens. Nat Neurosci 2010; 13: 1137-43.

[88]   Cedar H. DNA methylation and gene activity. Cell 1988; 53:3-4.

[89]   Razin A, Riggs AD. DNA methylation and gene function. Science 1980; 210: 604-10.

[90] Tamame M, Antequera F, Villanueva JR, Santos T. High-frequency conversion to a "fluffy" developmental phenotype in Aspergillus spp. by 5-azacytidine treatment: evidence for involvement of a single nuclear gene. Mol Cell Biol 1983; 3: 2287-97.

[91] Jugloff DG, Vandamme K, Logan R, Visanji NP, Brotchie JM, Eubanks JH. Targeted delivery of an Mecp2 transgene to forebrain neurons improves the behavior of female Mecp2-deficient mice. Hum Mol Genet 2008; 17: 1386-96.

[92] Luikenhuis S, Giacometti E, Beard CF, Jaenisch R. Expression of MeCP2 in postmitotic neurons rescues Rett syndrome in mice. Proc Natl Acad Sci U S A 2004; 101: 6033-8.

[93] Bontekoe CJ, McIlwain KL, Nieuwenhuizen IM, Yuva-Paylor LA, Nellis A, Willemsen R, *et al.* Knockout mouse model for Fxr2: a model for mental retardation. Hum Mol Genet 2002; 11: 487-98.

[94] Consortium TD-BFX. Fmr1 knockout mice: a model to study fragile X mental retardation. The Dutch-Belgian Fragile X Consortium. Cell 1994; 78: 23-33.

[95] Francis YI, Fa M, Ashraf H, Zhang H, Staniszewski A, Latchman DS, *et al.* Dysregulation of histone acetylation in the APP/PS1 mouse model of Alzheimer's disease. J Alzheimers Dis 2009; 18: 131-9.

[96] Feng J, Zhou Y, Campbell SL, Le T, Li E, Sweatt JD, *et al.* Dnmt1 and Dnmt3a maintain DNA methylation and regulate synaptic function in adult forebrain neurons. Nat Neurosci 2010; 13: 423-30.

[97] Weeber EJ, Beffert U, Jones C, Christian JM, Forster E, Sweatt JD, *et al.* Reelin and ApoE receptors cooperate to enhance hippocampal synaptic plasticity and learning. J Biol Chem 2002; 277: 39944-52.

[98] Lubin FD, Roth TL, Sweatt JD. Epigenetic regulation of BDNF gene transcription in the consolidation of fear memory. J Neurosci 2008; 28: 10576-86.

[99] Frankland PW, O'Brien C, Ohno M, Kirkwood A, Silva AJ. Alpha-CaMKII-dependent plasticity in the cortex is required for permanent memory. Nature 2001; 411: 309-13.

[100] Miller CA, Gavin CF, White JA, Parrish RR, Honasoge A, Yancey CR, *et al.* Cortical DNA methylation maintains remote memory. Nat Neurosci 2010; 13: 664-6.

[101] Day JJ, Sweatt JD. Cognitive neuroepigenetics: A role for epigenetic mechanisms in learning and memory. Neurobiol Learn Mem 2011; 96: 2-12.

[102] Beliavtseva LM, Kulikova OG, Razumovskaia NI, Borodkin Iu S. [Action of the memory stimulant etimizol on brain chromatin]. Dokl Akad Nauk SSSR 1985; 283: 490-2.

[103] Haggarty SJ, Tsai LH. Probing the role of HDACs and mechanisms of chromatin-mediated neuroplasticity. Neurobiol Learn Mem 2011; 96: 41-52.

[104] Guan JS, Haggarty SJ, Giacometti E, Dannenberg JH, Joseph N, Gao J, *et al.* HDAC2 negatively regulates memory formation and synaptic plasticity. Nature 2009; 459: 55-60.

[105] Alarcon JM, Malleret G, Touzani K, Vronskaya S, Ishii S, Kandel ER, *et al.* Chromatin acetylation, memory, and LTP are impaired in CBP+/- mice: a model for the cognitive deficit in Rubinstein-Taybi syndrome and its amelioration. Neuron 2004; 42: 947-59.

[106] Haggarty SJ, Tsai LH. Probing the role of HDACs and mechanisms of chromatin-mediated neuroplasticity. Neurobiol Learn Mem 2011; PMID 21545841

[107] Lin HY, Chen CS, Lin SP, Weng JR. Targeting histone deacetylase in cancer therapy. Med Res Rev 2006; 26: 397-413.

[108] Wagner JM, Hackanson B, Lubbert M, Jung M. Histone deacetylase (HDAC) inhibitors in recent clinical trials for cancer therapy. Clin Epigenetics 2010; 1: 117-36.

[109] Atadja PW. HDAC inhibitors and cancer therapy. Prog Drug Res 2011; 67: 175-95.

[110] Koshibu K, Graff J, Beullens M, Heitz FD, Berchtold D, Russig H, *et al.* Protein phosphatase 1 regulates the histone code for long-term memory. J Neurosci 2009; 29: 13079-89.

[111] Koshibu K, Graff J, Mansuy IM. Nuclear protein phosphatase-1: an epigenetic regulator of fear memory and amygdala long-term potentiation. Neuroscience 2011; 173: 30-6.

[112] Canettieri G, Morantte I, Guzman E, Asahara H, Herzig S, Anderson SD, *et al.* Attenuation of a phosphorylation-dependent activator by an HDAC-PP1 complex. Nat Struct Biol 2003; 10: 175-81.

[113] Murnion ME, Adams RR, Callister DM, Allis CD, Earnshaw WC, Swedlow JR. Chromatin-associated protein phosphatase 1 regulates aurora-B and histone H3 phosphorylation. J Biol Chem 2001; 276: 26656-65.

[114] Graff J, Koshibu K, Jouvenceau A, Dutar P, Mansuy IM. Protein phosphatase 1-dependent transcriptional programs for long-term memory and plasticity. Learn Mem 2010; 17: 355-63.

[115] Kandel ER. The molecular biology of memory storage: a dialogue between genes and synapses. Science 2001; 294: 1030-8.

[116] Guan Z, Giustetto M, Lomvardas S, Kim JH, Miniaci MC, Schwartz JH, *et al.* Integration of long-term-memory-related synaptic plasticity involves bidirectional regulation of gene expression and chromatin structure. Cell 2002; 111: 483-93.

[117] Chwang WB, O'Riordan KJ, Levenson JM, Sweatt JD. ERK/MAPK regulates hippocampal histone phosphorylation following contextual fear conditioning. Learn Mem 2006; 13: 322-8.

[118] Kim J, Krichevsky A, Grad Y, Hayes GD, Kosik KS, Church GM, *et al.* Identification of many microRNAs that copurify with polyribosomes in mammalian neurons. Proc Natl Acad Sci U S A 2004; 101: 360-5.

[119] Redondo RL, Morris RG. Making memories last: the synaptic tagging and capture hypothesis. Nat Rev Neurosci 2011; 12: 17-30.

[120] Swanger SA, Bassell GJ. Making and breaking synapses through local mRNA regulation. Curr Opin Genet Dev 2011; PMID 21530231.

[121] Yu JY, Chung KH, Deo M, Thompson RC, Turner DL. MicroRNA miR-124 regulates neurite outgrowth during neuronal differentiation. Exp Cell Res 2008 ; 314: 2618-33.

[122] Natera-Naranjo O, Aschrafi A, Gioio AE, Kaplan BB. Identification and quantitative analyses of microRNAs located in the distal axons of sympathetic neurons. RNA 2010; 16: 1516-29.

[123] Hengst U, Cox LJ, Macosko EZ, Jaffrey SR. Functional and selective RNA interference in developing axons and growth cones. J Neurosci 2006; 26: 5727-32.

[124] Krutzfeldt J, Kuwajima S, Braich R, Rajeev KG, Pena J, Tuschl T, *et al.* Specificity, duplex degradation and subcellular localization of antagomirs. Nucleic Acids Res 2007; 35: 2885-92.

[125] Shibata M, Nakao H, Kiyonari H, Abe T, Aizawa S. MicroRNA-9 regulates neurogenesis in mouse telencephalon by targeting multiple transcription factors. J Neurosci 2011; 31: 3407-22.

[126] Esau CC. Inhibition of microRNA with antisense oligonucleotides. Methods 2008; 44: 55-60.

[127] Rajasethupathy P, Fiumara F, Sheridan R, Betel D, Puthanveettil SV, Russo JJ, *et al.* Characterization of small RNAs in Aplysia reveals a role for miR-124 in constraining synaptic plasticity through CREB. Neuron 2009; 63: 803-17.

[128] Konopka W, Kiryk A, Novak M, Herwerth M, Parkitna JR, Wawrzyniak M, *et al.* MicroRNA loss enhances learning and memory in mice. J Neurosci 2010; 30: 14835-42.

[129] Gao J, Wang WY, Mao YW, Graff J, Guan JS, Pan L, *et al.* A novel pathway regulates memory and plasticity *via* SIRT1 and miR-134. Nature 2010; 466: 1105-9.

[130] Gaughwin P, Ciesla M, Yang H, Lim B, Brundin P. Stage-Specific Modulation of Cortical Neuronal Development by Mmu-miR-134. Cereb Cortex 2011; PMID 21228099

[131] Sajikumar S, Korte M. Metaplasticity governs compartmentalization of synaptic tagging and capture through brain-derived neurotrophic factor (BDNF) and protein kinase Mzeta (PKMzeta). Proc Natl Acad Sci U S A 2011; 108: 2551-6.

[132] Bredy TW, Lin Q, Wei W, Baker-Andresen D, Mattick JS. MicroRNA regulation of neural plasticity and memory. Neurobiol Learn Mem 2011; 96: 89-94.

[133] Redondo RL, Morris RG. Making memories last: the synaptic tagging and capture hypothesis. Nat Rev Neurosci 2011; 12: 17-30.

[134] Lugli G, Larson J, Martone ME, Jones Y, Smalheiser NR. Dicer and eIF2c are enriched at postsynaptic densities in adult mouse brain and are modified by neuronal activity in a calpain-dependent manner. J Neurochem 2005; 94: 896-905.

[135] Wibrand K, Panja D, Tiron A, Ofte ML, Skaftnesmo KO, Lee CS, *et al.* Differential regulation of mature and precursor microRNA expression by NMDA and metabotropic glutamate receptor activation during LTP in the adult dentate gyrus *in vivo.* Eur J Neurosci 2010; 31: 636-45.

[136] Ashraf SI, McLoon AL, Sclarsic SM, Kunes S. Synaptic protein synthesis associated with memory is regulated by the RISC pathway in Drosophila. Cell 2006; 124: 191-205.

[137] Tabolacci E, Pietrobono R, Moscato U, Oostra BA, Chiurazzi P, Neri G. Differential epigenetic modifications in the FMR1 gene of the fragile X syndrome after reactivating pharmacological treatments. Eur J Hum Genet 2005; 13: 641-8.

[138] Nomura T, Kimura M, Horii T, Morita S, Soejima H, Kudo S, *et al.* MeCP2-dependent repression of an imprinted miR-184 released by depolarization. Hum Mol Genet 2008; 17: 1192-9.

[139] Sakabe K, Wang Z, Hart GW. Beta-N-acetylglucosamine (O-GlcNAc) is part of the histone code. Proc Natl Acad Sci U S A 2010; 107: 19915-20.

[140] Tweedie-Cullen RY, Reck JM, Mansuy IM. Comprehensive mapping of post-translational modifications on synaptic, nuclear, and histone proteins in the adult mouse brain. J Proteome Res 2009; 8: 4966-82.

[141] Compte A. Computational and *in vitro* studies of persistent activity: edging towards cellular and synaptic mechanisms of working memory. Neuroscience 2006; 139: 135-51.

[142] Turing. Computing Machinery and Intelligence. Mind 1950; 54: 433-60.

[143] Mink WD, Best PJ, Olds J. Neurons in paradoxical sleep and motivated behavior. Science 1967; 158: 1335-6.

[144] Nader K, Schafe GE, Le Doux JE. Fear memories require protein synthesis in the amygdala for reconsolidation after retrieval. Nature 2000; 406: 722-6.

CHAPTER 3

Epigenetics of Stress

Andrew Collins, María Gutièrrez-Mecinas, Alexandra F. Trollope and Johannes M.H.M. Reul*

Henry Wellcome Laboratories for Integrative Neuroscience and Endocrinology, Dorothy Hodgkin Building, University of Bristol, Whitson Street, Bristol, BS1 3NY, United Kingdom

Abstract: Poor stress-coping is associated with a greater chance of developing a psychiatric illness such as post-traumatic stress disorder (PTSD) or depression. Lifestyle interventions which facilitate more appropriate responses to stress are much sought after. Exercise is one such intervention and is now commonly being prescribed as a co-treatment along with drugs for treating depression. Exercised rodents display reduced anxiety and impulsivity in a variety of behavioral paradigms. Rats exposed to psychological stress show differential epigenetic and gene expression mechanisms at the dentate gyrus (DG) after long-term voluntary exercise. Alterations within ERK MAPK signalling to chromatin seem to modulate the number of epigenetically marked neurons in the DG, improving cognitive responses to a stress-related event. Other lifestyle interventions such as nutrition or better maternal care in early life have been shown to induce changes at the epigenome which impact positively on mental health.

Keywords: Stress, brain, hippocampus, learning, memory, chromatin, histone, exercise, glucocorticoid hormone, HPA axis, dentate gyrus, ERK MAPK, MSK1, immediate early gene, PTSD, anxiety, depression, cognition, adaptation, early life experience, DNA methylation, c-Fos, Egr-1, social defeat, CREB.

3.1. INTRODUCTION

The ability to cope with stress is not just a modern phenomenon – it has aided our survival for millennia. On a daily basis, health practitioners and government adverts describe the medical problems associated with a stressful, sedentary lifestyle. Those who fail to manage stress in a pertinent manner or are subject to early life stress are more vulnerable to depression in their lifetime [1]. Other stress-related psychiatric illnesses such as post-traumatic stress disorder (PTSD) are disabling psychiatric disorders which affect millions worldwide. Any lifestyle

*Address correspondence to Johannes M.H.M. Reul: Henry Wellcome Laboratories for Integrative Neuroscience and Endocrinology, Dorothy Hodgkin Building, University of Bristol, Whitson Street, Bristol, BS1 3NY, United Kingdom; Tel: +44 117 331 3137; Email: Hans.Reul@bristol.ac.uk

Marcelina Párrizas, Rosa Gasa and Perla Kaliman (Eds)

intervention which enhances stress-coping would help alleviate this burden to society and to the individual. This chapter examines the putative epigenetic mechanisms underlying appropriate behavioral responses to stress. The effects of early life stress and maternal care, as well as the benefits of a nutritious diet, shall be discussed. The major theme, however, is the positive impact of exercise on stress-coping ability through distinct epigenetic mechanisms at the dentate gyrus, a subregion of the limbic structure hippocampus.

3.1.1. Stress & the HPA Axis

Central to a definition of stress is the maintenance of homeostasis; keeping a stable internal environment in the face of changing external conditions. The threat to homeostasis may be real or imaginary and it affects the organism at the physiological or psychological level [2]. The most immediate response to stress involves CNS-induced increases in arousal, vigilance, cognition, attention and aggression [3]. These changes arise through activation of the autonomic nervous system (ANS), particularly the sympathetic branch. Catecholamines are released into the blood leading to tachycardia, increased force of cardiac contraction, peripheral vasoconstriction and the mobilization of energy resources.

The endocrine component of the stress response is mediated by the hypothalamic-pituitary-adrenal (HPA) axis. This system originates with parvocellular neurons in the hypothalamic paraventricular nucleus (PVN). These neurons send projections to the median eminence where the neuropeptides corticotrophin-releasing factor (CRF) and vasopressin (AVP) are released that travel *via* the portal blood system to the anterior pituitary. At the pituitary, they stimulate the synthesis and release of adrenocorticotropic hormone (ACTH) into the blood stream which acts on the adrenal cortex to release glucocorticoid hormones [4].

Glucocorticoids (GCs; corticosterone in rats and mice, cortisol in humans) exert strong metabolic actions such as gluconeogenesis, mobilization of amino acids, fat breakdown or inhibition of glucose uptake in muscle; all of which serve to maintain normal blood glucose concentrations. GCs act at the cellular level *via* glucocorticoid (GR) receptors which are present in virtually all cells of the body. In the brain, GCs bind in addition to GRs also to mineralocorticoid receptors (MRs; [5, 6]. MRs have a ten-fold higher affinity for corticosterone than GRs and have been implicated in the appraisal and initiation of the stress response [7]. GRs become more activated at the peak of the circadian rhythm and during the stress response. GCs exert negative feedback actions at the PVN and anterior pituitary to inhibit the synthesis and release of CRF and ACTH, respectively. In addition to the termination of the stress response and the mobilization of energy resources for recovery, GCs *via* GRs also play an important role (amongst other functions) in the control of the immune system [8] and the consolidation of emotional and episodic memories of the stressful event [9-11].

3.2. MATERNAL LIFESTYLE IMPACTS ON HPA AXIS DEVELOPMENT *VIA* EPIGENETIC MECHANISMS

In 2004, Michael J. Meaney and colleagues presented evidence that maternal care could mediate long-term effects on gene expression in the offspring *via* stable alterations of DNA methylation and chromatin structure [12]. Previous evidence had shown that maternal behavior could result in HPA axis adaptations but the contribution in terms of epigenetic mechanisms putatively involved in such regulation was unknown [13]. Meaney and colleagues linked an increase of pup licking and grooming (LG) and arched back nursing (ABN) by rat mothers to an alteration of the offspring epigenome at the exon 1_7 of the glucocorticoid receptor gene promoter in the hippocampus. Adult offspring from a more maternally caring (high LG-ABN mothers) environment exhibited increased hippocampal GR expression and enhanced glucocorticoid feedback sensitivity. This apparently accounted for, to some degree, the more modest HPA responses to stress in offspring of high LG-ABN mothers.

In terms of epigenetics, the pattern of DNA methylation, histone acetylation and transcription factor binding at the GR promoter was found to be different between high- and low LG-ABN mothers. For example, regarding the EGR1 (also termed NGFI-A or ZIF268) response element, 5' CpG dinucleotides were demethylated in the high-, but not in the low-LG-ABN group. This difference in DNA methylation was associated with the level of maternal behavior during the first week of life. This work was seminal as it showed that epigenetic mechanisms mediate "environmental programming" which is reflected in gene expression changes in the offspring.

McGowan *et al.* [14] translated this work from a rat into a human context to further examine the epigenetic regulation of the HPA axis. They found epigenetic differences at the human GR promoter in post-mortem hippocampus tissue obtained from suicide victims with a history of childhood abuse and healthy controls. It had been known that childhood adversity is linked to aberrant HPA axis stress responses when adult and may result in a greater risk for many forms of psychopathology [15, 16]. Aberrant hippocampal GR expression has been associated with suicide, schizophrenia and other mood disorders [17, 18]. Thus, stressful environments such as that encountered by those with a history of childhood abuse can facilitate epigenetic modifications which may entail an increased risk to depression and/or suicide later in life. McGowan and colleagues found decreased hippocampal GR mRNA in post-mortem brains of those with a history of childhood abuse. They found a similar pattern of expression for the GR 1F splice variant. They observed an increased DNA methylation at the GR promoter which they believed would lead to decreased Egr1 binding to the promoter resulting in reduced GR gene transcription. Together, their work on rat and humans implicate epigenetic mechanisms in potentially influencing long-lasting HPA axis changes in the offspring with behavioral and psychopathological impact.

3.3. THE EPIGENETIC MECHANISMS BEHIND STRESS-RELATED PSYCHIATRIC DISORDERS

The study of epigenetics initially expanded in developmental and cancer biology where patterns of gene expression are passed on without alteration from parent to daughter cells. These initial studies aided the discovery and conceptualisation regarding the functional roles of chromatin remodelling and DNA modifications which are now fundamental to recent advances in the field of epigenetics. Long-lasting stable behavioral adaptations brought about by epigenetically-mediated gene expression changes are a suitable candidate for further investigation in psychiatric disorders. Depression is a relatively long-lasting and persistent disease and anti-depressant drug treatment takes several weeks to take effect. These two characteristics imply the need for stable alterations in gene expression which take time to develop but can become permanent. One treatment for depression, electroconvulsive shock (ECS), has been applied chronically to rats in an attempt to elucidate the role of epigenetic mechanisms underlying long-term adaptations in the hippocampus. It was found that chronic (but not acute) ECS upregulated both BDNF and CREB gene expression within the hippocampus. Observations in other studies corresponded with this finding and reported increased neurotrophic signalling (*e.g.* BDNF) which, according to the authors, mediated antidepressant activity [19, 20]. The histone modification events at distinct *bdnf* gene promoters were different depending on whether ECS treatment was chronic or acute. In particular, increased H3 acetylation was found at Bdnf promoters 3 and 4, along with increased expression of *Bdnf* transcripts after chronic ECS.

A chronic social defeat stress model [21] whereby a mouse is exposed to aggressive resident mice of the same strain has apparent similarities to symptoms of human depression. Experiments using such a model have reported long-lasting increases in dimethylation at histone H3K27 (*i.e.* lysine27 in histone H3) in the promoter region of *bdnf*. Such a histone modification is thought to be repressive and causes down-regulation of *bdnf* III and *bdnf* IV splice variants within the hippocampus. Chronic treatment with the antidepressant imipramine reverses the repression of the *bdnf* gene by inducing transcription activating histone modifications such as histone H3 acetylation and H3K4 methylation at the gene promoter. This reversal of repression is believed to occur through down-regulation of HDAC (histone de-acetylase) expression in the hippocampus of animals subject to chronic social defeat [20].

Other studies reveal extensive histone H3K4 methylation by a class of antidepressants called monoamine oxidase inhibitors and subsequent long-term transcriptional regulation [22]. Such long-lasting stable neuronal adaptations brought about by histone modifications are often located in the hippocampus and are thought to underlie long-term changes in behavior. Further examination of the roles of these chromatin remodelling events and their induction by specific HDAC, HMT (histone methyl transferase) and HDM (histone de-methylase) inhibitors could prove effective in the search for antidepressant treatments [23].

3.4. STRESS LEAVES ITS (EPIGENETIC) MARK ON THE DENTATE GYRUS

3.4.1. *In vitro* Evidence of Epigenetic Control of Gene Expression Extends to *in vivo* Stress Paradigms

For many years now, our laboratory has sought to shed light on the precise molecular machinery confined to stress-related memory formation. This section details the short history of *in vitro* and *in vivo* discoveries which crystallised the concept that an interaction between glucocorticoids and the ERK MAPK cascade (activated by the NMDA receptor) enable the distinct epigenetic marks in dentate gyrus granule neurons which are involved in the formation of enduring memories of significant events.

As already discussed in Chapter 1, covalent modifications of histone molecules are an example of an epigenetic mechanism which can impact on chromatin structure and determine its functional state. That such a state could facilitate gene transcription was alluded to with *in vitro* experiments conducted by Clayton and colleagues [24]. They employed chromatin immunoprecipitation (ChIP) techniques to show that a double modification (phosphorylation of Serine-10 combined with acetylation of Lysine-14 (H3S10p-K14ac)) invoked the nucleosomal response required for immediate early gene (IEG) activation. Indeed, H3S10p-K14ac is instrumental in the local opening of condensed, inactive chromatin and as such could mediate transcriptional activation of dormant genes.

By the end of the 1990s, the serendipitous discovery of H3S10p-K14ac-positive neurons in the dentate gyrus of rats and mice expanded this work to *in vivo* models [25]. We were interested in how animals adapt to and learn from psychologically stressful challenges. Using antibodies that specifically recognized the dual histone mark, we uncovered a speckled nuclear immuno-staining pattern in nuclei of sparsely distributed DG neurons. When rats or mice were confronted with a single psychological challenge such as forced swimming, a predator or a novel environment, the number of H3S10p-K14ac-positive neurons increased specifically in the dentate gyrus and remained elevated for up to 4 hours [26-28]. A similar dentate gyrus response pattern was observed after Morris water maze learning and fear conditioning suggesting that these epigenetic changes contribute to neuroplastic mechanisms which mediate learning and memory processes (Chandramohan and Reul, unpublished observations). David Sweatt and colleagues found histone H3 phosphorylation and acetylation in hippocampal extracts when studying these learning and memory paradigms [29].

In terms of IEG gene activation, we showed that the dual H3S10p-K14ac epigenetic marks facilitate induction of *c-fos in vivo* [27, 28, 30]. To arrive at this discovery, we first observed parallel increases of H3S10p-K14ac- and C-FOS-immuno-positive neurons amongst dentate granule cells after psychological stress in rats and mice. Co-localisation of the epigenetic mark and gene product in immuno-fluorescent studies followed before ChIP and qPCR techniques confirmed that H3S10p-K14ac marks occur in the *c-fos* promoter region in dentate gyrus neurons [30] (A.F. Trollope and J.M.H.M. Reul, unpublished observations). The phospho-acetylation of histone H3 associated with *c-Fos* induction after psychological challenges (*e.g.* forced swimming, novelty) was confined to the dentate gyrus specifically and alludes to different epigenetic mechanisms activating gene expression at other brain regions.

3.4.2. What is the Identity of the Cascade which Signals to Chromatin within the DG to give H3S10pK14ac?

A combination of extracellular and intracellular signalling pathways is required to link environmental stimuli with the necessary epigenetic apparatus to invoke an appropriate behavioral response and memory formation. In extracellular terms, both glucocorticoids and glutamate were found to be essential [26-28] for the forced swimming and novelty-induced histone H3 phospho-acetylation and *c-fos* induction at the dentate gyrus. Dual activation of these pathways was essential [27] and a role of mineralocorticoid receptors and nitric oxide in mediation of this activation was excluded [27, 28].The involvement of the intracellular ERK MAPK cascade in histone H3 phospho-acetylation was not surprising given the purported role of this signalling pathway in memory formation [31]. Pharmacological and gene deletion approaches identified the involvement of extracellular signal-regulated kinases ERK1/2 and the mitogen-and stress activated kinases 1 and 2 (MSK1/2; [28]). A combination of immunohistochemical and immunofluorescence studies showed the localization of pERK1/2 and pMSK1 in sparse dentate granule neurons. Furthermore, co-localization of pERK1/2, pMSK1 and H3S10p-K14ac within the very same neuron was demonstrated after swim stress (see Fig. **1**; [30]) (Gutierrez-Mecinas *et al.* submitted).

Once activated, MSK1 has a kinase function at H3S10 and CREB and thus may explain one of the modifications of histone H3. Bilang-Bleuel *et al.* [26] previously showed an enhanced phosphorylation of CREB in dentate gyrus

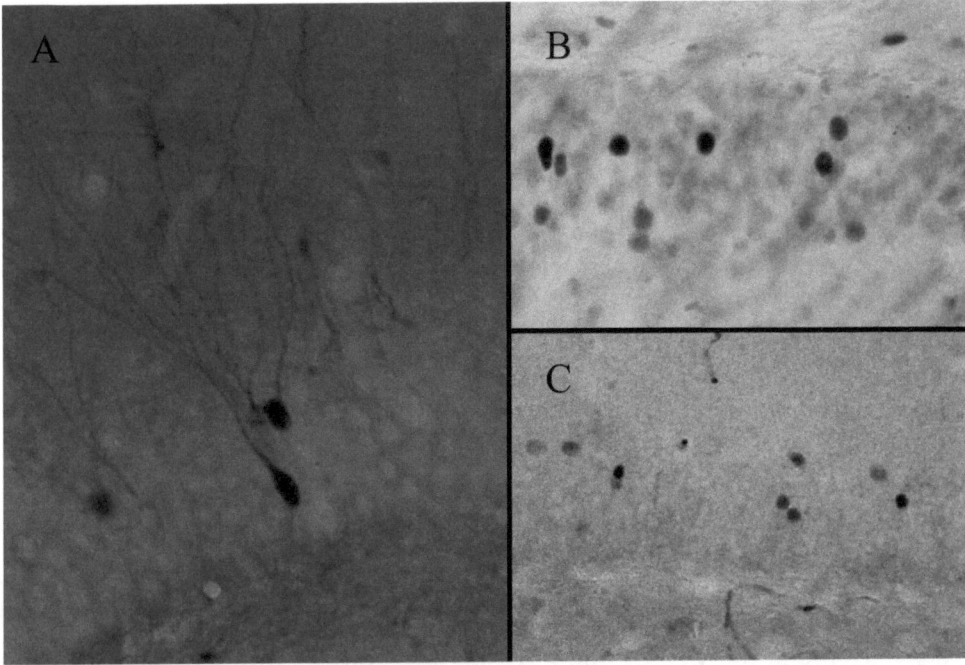

Figure 1: Representative images of the granular cell layer of the rat dentate gyrus showing immunoreactivity of pERK1/2 (A), pMSK1 (B), and C-FOS (C) after 15min of forced swimming. pERK1/2-IR is present in the cell body and dendrites whilst pMSK1- and C-FOS-IR is confined to the nucleus. Images were taken at 40x magnification.

neurons after forced swimming. The *c-fos* promoter contains a CRE site to which pCREB dimers can bind and exert transactivational stimulation of gene transcription. Furthermore, pCREB is able to recruit CBP/p300 (which has histone acetyl-transferase (HAT) activity) to the promoter [32]. However, CREB is ubiquitously phosphorylated in nearly all dentate gyrus neurons after forced swimming [33] which is in contrast to the sparsely populated H3S10p-K14ac-positive neurons. Therefore the role of pCREB in the dentate gyrus may be more generalised such as in neuroprotection and not specific to stress [34]. A protein which could play a distinct role in acetylating the H3S10p at the *c-fos* promoter is the E twenty-six (ETS)-domain containing protein Elk-1 (Ets-like protein 1) [35-37] which has been shown *in vitro* to be activated through the ERK MAPK pathway. Similar to pCREB, ELK1 can recruit p300 to the promoter but it does so by binding to the ELK-1 binding site at the serum response element (SRE) within the *c-fos* promoter. Immuno-fluorescent studies showing co-localisation of pELK-1, pERK1/2, pMSK1, H3S10p-K14ac and C-FOS within the same dentate gyrus neurons after forced swimming serve to bolster their respective roles in the chromatin remodelling event (Gutierrez-Mecinas *et al.* submitted).

Our postulated pathway leading to chromatin remodelling in distinct dentate gyrus granule neurons requires dual activation of both GR- and NMDA receptor-mediated signalling. The precise mechanism of action of GR is currently unclear. GRs do not have any enzyme activity to phosphorylate or acetylate histone molecules directly. *In vitro* work has shown that GRs may be required for recruiting chromatin-remodeling complexes and histone modifying enzymes to the chromatin [38-40]. Recently, we postulated that since both GR and NMDA receptor activation are required for downstream epigenetic and gene expression effects, GRs may be acting through a direct interaction with NMDA receptor-activated signaling molecules of the ERK MAPK pathway. We indeed found that pERK1/2 requires activated GRs in order to facilitate phosphorylation of MSK1 and ELK-1 in dentate granule neurons [30]. Levels of pERK1/2, pMSK1 and pElk-1 were found to peak 15 min after stress before returning to baseline at 1 h. This activation of ERK MAPK is quicker than that found previously in an *in vitro* study. Revest *et al.* [41] treated AtT-20 cells with glucocorticoid hormone and found increased Ras, Raf-1, ERK1/2 and pERK1/2 levels after 1-3 hours. The slower effects of glucocorticoid on ERK MAPK signalling in the pituitary cell line suggests a different process to that occurring with DG granule cell neurons. Further work is presently undertaken to determine the precise mechanisms underlying the interaction of GRs with NMDA receptor-activated ERK MAPK/MSK1-ELK-1 signalling pathway and its implications for chromatin modifications, gene expression and the consolidation of behavioral responses.

3.4.3. Exercise-Induced Epigenetic Mechanisms at the Dentate Gyrus Facilitate Improved Stress-Coping and Cognition

Evidence has been accumulating which underscores the idea that exercise is beneficial for the brain. In addition to the positive effects exerted on the cardiovascular system [42], the immune system [43] or in combating obesity [44], regular exercise is now frequently linked to enhancement of cognition or as neuroprotection against neurodegeneration [45, 46]. Psychiatrists promote the benefits of a lifestyle which includes regular exercise and they prescribe it as a co-treatment along with drugs for treating depression and anxiety disorders [47-49].

For a number of years, we have used a voluntary wheel-running paradigm with rodents to investigate the impact of long-term voluntary exercise. Droste *et al.* [50] initially found that 4 weeks of voluntary exercise (4 km per day on average) in mice led to less abdominal fat, lighter thymuses and heavier adrenal glands than sedentary controls. Adaptations to the HPA axis of exercised animals enable more pertinent responses to the type of stress presented. After a forced swimming challenge, for example, exercised animals showed almost double the level of corticosterone as controls. After novelty stress however the glucocorticoid response in the exercised animals was much lower than that in the control animals [50, 51]. Interestingly, when the responses in free corticosterone were examined [by a method called *in vivo* microdialysis] no differences between exercised and sedentary rats were found using either stressor [52]. Currently, the reasons for the discrepancy between the findings on total and free corticosterone responses are unknown. Sleep/EEG recordings by Lancel *et al.* [53] in freely behaving exercising and sedentary mice showed that overall exercise leads to improved sleep quality because it enhances sleep continuity, increases slow-wave sleep and decreases REM sleep. In terms of stress-coping, numerous experiments have shown that exercise leads to reduced anxiety [47, 48, 54]. In the open field test, modified hole board, elevated plus maze and light-dark box, exercised animals show reduced impulsivity and less anxiety than sedentary controls [54].

More recently, studies have linked improved stress-coping after exercise with distinct epigenetic and gene expression mechanisms at the dentate gyrus. Exposure to a novel environment is a mild psychological stress which has previously been shown to evoke lower corticosterone responses from exercised rats than sedentary controls [50]. Collins *et al.* [55] found that exercised animals were less anxious than sedentary controls in a novel environment. By the end of the 30 min exposure, exercised rats displayed similar behavior to resting conditions in the home cage, *i.e.* lying and sleeping behavior. Sedentary control rats, however, continued to investigate their surroundings, apparently anxious and vigilant (see Fig. **2**).

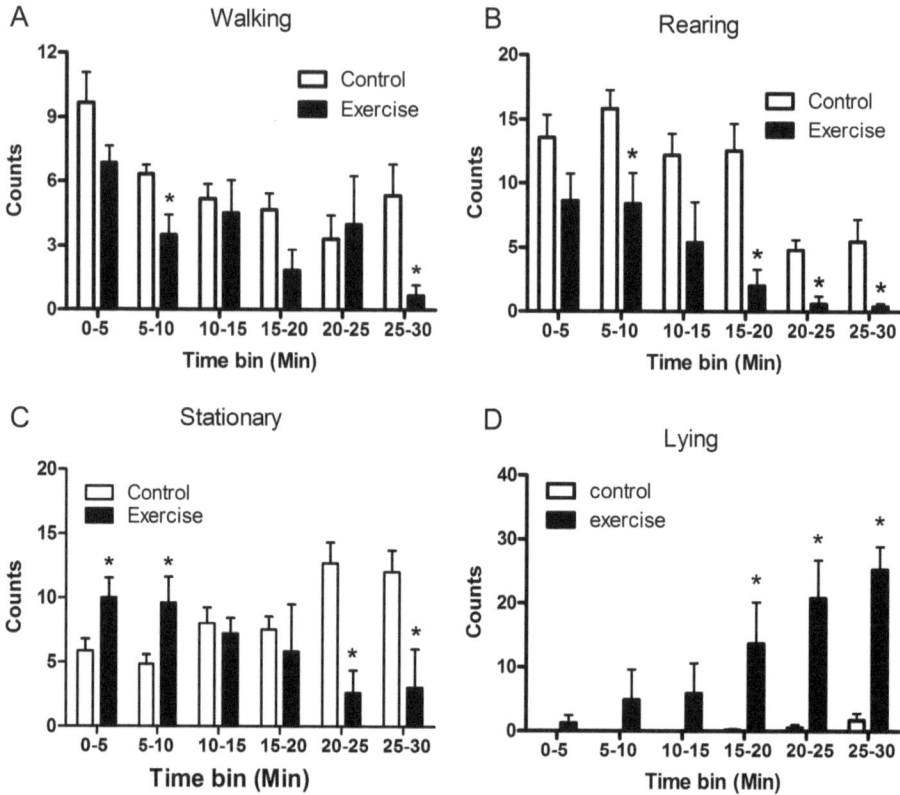

Figure 2: Behavior of control and exercised rats during exposure to a novel environment, *i.e.* a new cage in a brightly lit (500 lx) room. Changes in walking (A), rearing (B), stationary (C) and lying behavior (D) were scored every 10 sec throughout the 30-min novelty exposure. Data were binned in 5-min time bins and expressed as behavioral counts (mean ± SEM, n=6). Statistical analyses: Two-way ANOVA with repeated measures: A, Effect of time: $F(5,45)=5.387$, $P=0.001$, Effect of exercise: $(F1,9)=4.739$, $P=0.057$, Interaction time x exercise: $F(5,45)=1.331$, not significant; B, Effect of time: $F(5,45)=15.545$, $P<0.0005$, Effect of exercise: $F(1,9)=14.263$, $P=0.004$, Interaction time x exercise: $F(5,45)=1.305$, not significant; C, Effect of time: $F(5,45)=0.153$, not significant, Effect of exercise: $F(1,9)=1.878$, not significant, Interaction time x exercise: $F(5,45)=7.881$, $P<0.0005$; D, Effect of time: $F(5,45)=11.529$, $P<0.0005$, Effect of exercise: $F(1,9)=11.332$, $P=0.008$, Interaction time x exercise: $F(5,45)=9.130$, $P<0.0005$.*, $P<0.05$, Student's t-test. Figure was taken from Collins *et al.* (2009) PLoS One 4: e4330.

Our ability to adapt to stressful events previously encountered is critical for our health and survival. Victims of severe trauma often respond in an exaggerated and maladaptive manner to sensory stimuli reminiscent of the initial stressful event. Post-traumatic stress disorder (PTSD) is a severe debilitating anxiety disorder and highlights how crucial it is that stress-related memory formation is allied with appropriate behavioral responses. When subjected to a forced swim test exercised and sedentary rats show similar behavior, *i.e.* predominantly struggling (climbing) or swimming behavior. However, in the forced swim re-test, exercised rats show an improved stress-coping behavioral response, compared with non-exercising controls. They remember better from the previous day's test that they cannot escape from the beaker and thus display much more an immobile posture, floating in the water with minimal movement. This is considered to be an adaptive response because it helps to conserve energy thereby increasing the chance of survival. At the molecular level in the brain, the immobility response has been shown to correlate highly with the expression of the dual H3S10p-K14ac epigenetic marks and *c-fos* induction at the dentate gyrus [11, 26, 28]. Interruption of the ERK MAPK cascade which signals to the chromatin results in abolition of the adaptive behavioral response. Exercised rats demonstrate differential epigenetic (H3S10p-K14ac) and gene expression (*c-fos*) within the dentate gyrus which may participate in the improved cognition and stress-coping observed in these animals [55].

3.4.4. Pharmacological Manipulation of H3S10p-K14ac Marks at the Dentate Gyrus

There is evidence suggesting that the hippocampus exerts an inhibitory tone on the activity of the HPA axis [5, 6, 56]. Hippocampal excitatory projections stimulate GABAergic neurons in the bed nucleus stria terminalis (BNST) which send projections to the PVN, inhibiting parvocellular neurons [56]. The hippocampus has been studied extensively with regards to its multi-faceted roles in episodic (contextual) memory formation, spatial navigation and the behavioral response to stress. The dentate gyrus plays a critical role in such processes by acting as a gateway; receiving inputs from the entorhinal cortex before processing this information and relaying it to other hippocampal regions. Here, the information is then integrated together with other relevant, stimulus-specific information to permit pertinent physiological and behavioral responses along with mnemonic-encoding of the event [57, 58]. The activation of dentate granule cells is sparse and limited to less than 5 % of the total granule cell population. It has been suggested that this relatively small activation is due to the strong tonic inhibition of the granule cells stemming from GABAergic interneurons [57, 58].

Through pharmacological approaches it is possible to modulate the level of inhibition to the granule cell layer; GABA-A agonists increase the tonic inhibition whilst inverse agonism at the same receptor attenuates inhibition. This approach was used by us [59] to show that the underlying GABAergic tone to the DG determines the number of dentate granule neurons expressing the dual H3S10p-K14ac epigenetic marks and associated *c-fos* induction after stress. Increasing the underlying GABAergic tone by administering the benzodiazepine, Lorazepam resulted in attenuated numbers of H3S10pK14ac- and C-FOS-positive neurons within the DG after a novelty challenge. In terms of behavior, Lorazepam-injected animals displayed reduced anxiety as would be expected. On the other hand, when GABAergic inhibition of the DG granule cells was reduced by FG7142 (partial inverse agonist at GABA-A receptor), greater numbers of both H3S10pK14ac- and C-FOS-positive neurons were found. Rats injected with FG7142 showed more anxious behavior in the novel environment [59]. These findings reveal that the prevailing anxiety state of the animal is reflected in the magnitude of H3S10pK14ac and C-FOS responses in the DG. In turn, how does the underlying ERK MAPK signalling to chromatin orchestrate differential epigenetic and gene expression responses at the DG?

Our recent investigation has shed light on the influence of altered ERK MAPK signalling within the DG after long-term exercise (Collins *et al.* (unpublished observations)). Exercised rats were shown to display reduced anxiety as well as differential epigenetic and gene expression response patterns to stress. We found attenuated levels of pERK1/2 and pMSK1 within mature DG neurons which correlated with reduced C-FOS expression and lowered anxiety behavior. The reduced ERK MAPK signalling may be due to changes in GABAergic neurotransmission as we found that exercise results in increased GABA synthesis capacity and modifications in GABA-A receptor subunit composition in the dentate gyrus [60]. Taken together, it appears that exercise modifies the signalling cascade behind the DG chromatin remodelling event which is involved in stress-related memory formation. As a lifestyle intervention, exercise can impact positively on the epigenome to mediate beneficial cognitive and anxiety responses in the face of stress.

3.5. EPIGENETIC MODIFICATIONS WITHIN HUMAN SKELETAL MUSCLE AFTER EXERCISE

Work has begun to establish the impact of epigenetic mechanisms in gene expression changes following exercise in human skeletal muscle. McGee *et al.* [61] examined global histone modifications which underlie exercise-induced chromatin remodelling and transcription in skeletal muscle. After one hour of cycling, global levels of acetylation at lysine residue 36 of histone H3 (H3K36ac) were increased. This particular modification has been associated with transcriptional elongation [62], involving initiation by RNA polymerase II. Interestingly, the McGee study did not observe an elevation in H3K9/14 acetylation globally after exercise. The prevailing acetylation state of histones is dictated by the balance between histone-acetyl-transferase (HAT) and histone deacetylase (HDAC) activities [63]. Therefore, the authors went on to examine the regulation of class IIa HDACs, enzymes that suppress histone acetylation. This class of enzymes does not possess any intrinsic HDAC themselves but can act as a scaffold to recruit a complex containing HDAC3 which have this function to particular promoters [64]. Overall, McGee *et al.* [61] found no difference in HDAC activity after exercise compared to resting levels. However, they did uncover differential subcellular localisation of the class IIa HDAC isoforms HDAC4 and HDAC5. These isoforms were found to undergo phosphorylation-dependent nuclear export, by AMP-activated protein kinase (AMPK) and CAMKII and thus removing their suppression of histone acetylation. Many of the benefits of aerobic exercise result from adaptations to the highly plastic skeletal muscle tissue. Distinct epigenetic mechanisms confer changes in gene expression within the skeletal muscle and nuclear export of histone-modifying enzymes appears to play an important role in these mechanisms.

3.6. NUTRITIONAL INTERVENTION IMPACTS ON THE EPIGENOME, ENABLING THE PERSONALISATION OF THERAPEUTIC APPROACHES

Nutrigenomics has been defined as the study of how nutrients impact on the (epi)genome. Included within this framework is "nutrigenetics" which aims to uncover the effect of individual genetic variation on the interaction between diet and disease [65]. Dieticians are striving to tailor nutritional advice for each individual, taking into account their own unique epigenome. Indeed, some epigenetic marks have recently been identified as biomarkers for obesity-related parameters.

Effective management of weight-loss programs are relevant given the global burden of obesity. After weight loss, various nutrient, neuronal and endocrine responses act to signal an "energy deficit". A number of metabolic adaptations then initiate which result in rapid weight gain in some people after a successful weight loss regime. This propensity to regain weight is different from person to person. Epigenetic marks had previously been known to be good indicators for the likelihood of this weight gain [66, 67]. Obesity predisposition, blood pressure and lipid profile have all been linked with certain epigenetic marks. Milagro *et al.* [68] compared patterns of DNA methylation between high and low responders to a hypocaloric diet. Microarray studies revealed 1034 CpGs differentially methylated between men who regained weight after weight loss and those who did not. Further examination of their results showed hypomethylation of several CpGs located in the promoter region of the ATP10A gene in high-responders before the dietary intervention. ATP10A encodes for an ATPase transporter which regulates lipid trafficking, fluidity of the plasma membrane and modulation of body fat [69]. ATP10A knockout mice are used as a model of obesity since they demonstrate an anabolic metabolism consistent with clinical features of obesity. This is therefore a useful biomarker and an early indication of aberrant responses to the metabolic effects of the weight loss program. Individual variability of the so called "epigenetic landscape" could be used to tailor dietary regimes for one specific epigenome as opposed to a "one size fits all" approach.

CONCLUSIONS

This chapter has highlighted how lifestyle choices influence our health and well-being from the womb to the grave. Decisions regarding diet and exercise partly determine our prevailing mood and ultimately impact upon our mental health. Our lab has demonstrated that distinct epigenetic mechanisms at the dentate gyrus may be molecular substrates for reduced anxiety, and improved stress-coping and cognition after exercise. It seems that regular activity tunes the epigenetic machinery to control genomic responses underlying neuroplasticity and cognitive changes in the face of stressful challenges. Although the precise nature of these effects is unclear at present, insights into epigenetic mechanisms could one day allow tailored medical and lifestyle interventions to suit our individual needs.

REFERENCES

[1]   Charney DS, Manji HK. Life stress, genes, and depression: multiple pathways lead to increased risk and new opportunities for intervention. Sci STKE 2004; 2004:re5.

[2]   McEwen BS. Mood disorders and allostatic load. Biol Psychiatry 2003; 54:200-207.

[3]   Chrousos GP. Stress and disorders of the stress system. Nat Rev Endocrinol 2009; 5:374-381.

[4]   Ulrich-Lai YM, Herman JP. Neural regulation of endocrine and autonomic stress responses. Nat Rev Neurosci 2009; 10:397-409.

[5]   Reul JMHM, de Kloet ER. Two receptor systems for corticosterone in rat brain: microdistribution and differential occupation. Endocrinology 1985; 117:2505-2511.

[6]   Reul JMHM, van den Bosch FR, de Kloet ER. Relative occupation of type-I and type-II corticosteroid receptors in rat brain following stress and dexamethasone treatment: functional implications. J Endocrinol 1987; 115:459-467.

[7]   de Kloet ER, Vreugdenhil E, Oitzl MS, Joels M. Brain corticosteroid receptor balance in health and disease. Endocr Rev 1998; 19:269-301.

[8]   Wiegers GJ, Reul JMHM. Induction of cytokine receptors by glucocorticoids: functional and pathological significance. Trends Pharmacol Sci 1998; 19:317-321.

[9]   de Kloet ER, Oitzl MS, Joels M. Stress and cognition: are corticosteroids good or bad guys? Trends Neurosci 1999; 22:422-426.

[10]   Smeets T, Wolf OT, Giesbrecht T, Sijstermans K, Telgen S, Joels M. Stress selectively and lastingly promotes learning of context-related high arousing information. Psychoneuroendocrinology 2009; 34:1152-1161.

[11]   Reul JMHM, Hesketh SA, Collins A, Mecinas MG. Epigenetic mechanisms in the dentate gyrus act as a molecular switch in hippocampus-associated memory formation. Epigenetics 2009; 4:434-439.

[12]   Weaver IC, Cervoni N, Champagne FA, D'Alessio AC, Sharma S, Seckl JR et al. Epigenetic programming by maternal behavior. Nat Neurosci 2004; 7:847-854.

[13]   Agrawal AA. Phenotypic plasticity in the interactions and evolution of species. Science 2001; 294:321-326.

[14]   McGowan PO, Sasaki A, D'Alessio AC, Dymov S, Labonte B, Szyf M et al. Epigenetic regulation of the glucocorticoid receptor in human brain associates with childhood abuse. Nat Neurosci 2009; 12(3):342-348.

[15]   Heim C, Nemeroff CB. The role of childhood trauma in the neurobiology of mood and anxiety disorders: preclinical and clinical studies. Biol Psychiatry 2001; 49:1023-1039.

[16]   Pruessner JC, Champagne F, Meaney MJ, Dagher A. Dopamine release in response to a psychological stress in humans and its relationship to early life maternal care: a positron emission tomography study using [11C]raclopride. J Neurosci 2004; 24:2825-2831.

[17]   Schatzberg AF, Rothschild AJ, Langlais PJ, Bird ED, Cole JO. A corticosteroid/dopamine hypothesis for psychotic depression and related states. J Psychiatr Res 1985; 19:57-64.

[18] Isometsa ET, Henriksson MM, Aro HM, Heikkinen ME, Kuoppasalmi KI, Lonnqvist JK. Suicide in major depression. Am J Psychiatry 1994; 151:530-536.

[19] Monteggia LM, Luikart B, Barrot M, Theobold D, Malkovska I, Nef S *et al.* Brain-derived neurotrophic factor conditional knockouts show gender differences in depression-related behaviors. Biol Psychiatry 2007; 61:187-197.

[20] Tsankova NM, Berton O, Renthal W, Kumar A, Neve RL, Nestler EJ. Sustained hippocampal chromatin regulation in a mouse model of depression and antidepressant action. Nat Neurosci 2006; 9:519-525.

[21] Berton O, McClung CA, Dileone RJ, Krishnan V, Renthal W, Russo SJ *et al.* Essential role of BDNF in the mesolimbic dopamine pathway in social defeat stress. Science 2006; 311:864-868.

[22] Lee MG, Wynder C, Schmidt DM, McCafferty DG, Shiekhattar R. Histone H3 lysine 4 demethylation is a target of nonselective antidepressive medications. Chem Biol 2006; 13:563-567.

[23] McClung CA, Ulery PG, Perrotti LI, Zachariou V, Berton O, Nestler EJ. DeltaFosB: a molecular switch for long-term adaptation in the brain. Brain Res Mol Brain Res 2004; 132:146-154.

[24] Clayton AL, Rose S, Barratt MJ, Mahadevan LC. Phosphoacetylation of histone H3 on c-fos- and c-jun-associated nucleosomes upon gene activation. EMBO J 2000; 19:3714-3726.

[25] Bilang-Bleuel A, Droste SK, Gesing A, Rech J, Linthorst ACE, Reul JMHM. Impact of stress and voluntary exercise on neurogenesis in the adult hippocampus: quantitative analysis by detection of Ki-67. Program No. 571.13. 2000 Neuroscience Meeting Planner. New Orleans, LA: Society for Neuroscience, 2000. Online.

[26] Bilang-Bleuel A, Ulbricht S, Chandramohan Y, De CS, Droste SK, Reul JMHM. Psychological stress increases histone H3 phosphorylation in adult dentate gyrus granule neurons: involvement in a glucocorticoid receptor-dependent behavioural response. Eur J Neurosci 2005; 22:1691-1700.

[27] Chandramohan Y, Droste SK, Reul JMHM. Novelty stress induces phospho-acetylation of histone H3 in rat dentate gyrus granule neurons through coincident signalling *via* the N-methyl-D-aspartate receptor and the glucocorticoid receptor: relevance for c-fos induction. J Neurochem 2007; 101:815-828.

[28] Chandramohan Y, Droste SK, Arthur JS, Reul JMHM. The forced swimming-induced behavioural immobility response involves histone H3 phospho-acetylation and c-Fos induction in dentate gyrus granule neurons *via* activation of the N-methyl-D-aspartate/extracellular signal-regulated kinase/mitogen- and stress-activated kinase signalling pathway. Eur J Neurosci 2008; 27:2701-2713.

[29] Chwang WB, Arthur JS, Schumacher A, Sweatt JD. The nuclear kinase mitogen- and stress-activated protein kinase 1 regulates hippocampal chromatin remodeling in memory formation. J Neurosci 2007; 27(46):12732-12742.

[30] Gutièrrez-Mecinas M, Collins A, Qian X, Hesketh SA, Reul JMHM. Forced swimming-evoked histone H3 phospho-acetylation and c-Fos induction in dentate gyrus granule neurons involves ERK1/2-mediated MSK1 and Elk-1 phosphorylation. Program No. 777.17. 2009 Neuroscience Meeting Planner. Chicago, IL: Society for Neuroscience, 2009. Online.

[31] Levenson JM, Sweatt JD. Epigenetic mechanisms in memory formation. Nat Rev Neurosci 2005; 6:108-118.

[32] Schiltz RL, Mizzen CA, Vassilev A, Cook RG, Allis CD, Nakatani Y. Overlapping but distinct patterns of histone acetylation by the human coactivators p300 and PCAF within nucleosomal substrates. J Biol Chem 1999; 274:1189-1192.

[33] Bilang-Bleuel A, Rech J, De CS, Holsboer F, Reul JMHM. Forced swimming evokes a biphasic response in CREB phosphorylation in extrahypothalamic limbic and neocortical brain structures in the rat. Eur J Neurosci 2002; 15:1048-1060.

[34] Papadia S, Stevenson P, Hardingham NR, Bading H, Hardingham GE. Nuclear Ca2+ and the cAMP response element-binding protein family mediate a late phase of activity-dependent neuroprotection. J Neurosci 2005; 25:4279-4287.

[35] Sharrocks AD. The ETS-domain transcription factor family. Nat Rev Mol Cell Biol 2001; 2:827-837.

[36] Yordy JS, Muise-Helmericks RC. Signal transduction and the Ets family of transcription factors. Oncogene 2000; 19:6503-6513.

[37] Shaw PE, Saxton J. Ternary complex factors: prime nuclear targets for mitogen-activated protein kinases. Int J Biochem Cell Biol 2003; 35:1210-1226.

[38] Li X, Wong J, Tsai SY, Tsai MJ, O'Malley BW. Progesterone and glucocorticoid receptors recruit distinct coactivator complexes and promote distinct patterns of local chromatin modification. Mol Cell Biol 2003; 23:3763-3773.

[39] Hebbar PB, Archer TK. Chromatin remodeling by nuclear receptors. Chromosoma 2003; 111:495-504.

[40] Kinyamu HK, Archer TK. Modifying chromatin to permit steroid hormone receptor-dependent transcription. Biochim Biophys Acta 2004; 1677:30-45.

[41] Revest JM, Di Blasi F, Kitchener P, Rouge-Pont F, Desmedt A, Turiault M *et al.* The MAPK pathway and Egr-1 mediate stress-related behavioral effects of glucocorticoids. Nat Neurosci 2005; 8:664-672.

[42] Kramer JM, Plowey ED, Beatty JA, Little HR, Waldrop TG. Hypothalamus, hypertension, and exercise. Brain Res Bull 2000; 53:77-85.

[43] Pedersen BK, Hoffman-Goetz L. Exercise and the immune system: regulation, integration, and adaptation. Physiol Rev 2000; 80:1055-1081.

[44] Friedman JE, Ferrara CM, Aulak KS, Hatzoglou M, McCune SA, Park S *et al.* Exercise training down-regulates ob gene expression in the genetically obese SHHF/Mcc-fa(cp) rat. Horm Metab Res 1997; 29:214-219.

[45] Creer DJ, Romberg C, Saksida LM, van Praag H, Bussey TJ. Running enhances spatial pattern separation in mice. Proc Natl Acad Sci U S A 2010; 107:2367-2372.

[46] O'Callaghan RM, Griffin EW, Kelly AM. Long-term treadmill exposure protects against age-related neurodegenerative change in the rat hippocampus. Hippocampus 2009; 19:1019-1029.

[47] Strohle A. Physical activity, exercise, depression and anxiety disorders. J Neural Transm 2009; 116:777-784.

[48] Steptoe A, Edwards S, Moses J, Mathews A. The effects of exercise training on mood and perceived coping ability in anxious adults from the general population. J Psychosom Res 1989; 33:537-547.

[49] Guszkowska M. [Effects of exercise on anxiety, depression and mood. Psychiatr Pol 2004; 38:611-620.

[50] Droste SK, Gesing A, Ulbricht S, Muller MB, Linthorst AC, Reul JMHM. Effects of long-term voluntary exercise on the mouse hypothalamic-pituitary-adrenocortical axis. Endocrinology 2003; 144:3012-3023.

[51]   Droste SK, Chandramohan Y, Hill LE, Linthorst AC, Reul JMHM. Voluntary exercise impacts on the rat hypothalamic-pituitary-adrenocortical axis mainly at the adrenal level. Neuroendocrinology 2007; 86:26-37.

[52]   Droste SK, Collins A, Lightman SL, Linthorst AC, Reul JMHM. Distinct, time-dependent effects of voluntary exercise on circadian and ultradian rhythms and stress responses of free corticosterone in the rat hippocampus. Endocrinology 2009; 150:4170-4179.

[53]   Lancel M, Droste SK, Sommer S, Reul JMHM. Influence of regular voluntary exercise on spontaneous and social stress-affected sleep in mice. Eur J Neurosci 2003; 17:2171-2179.

[54]   Binder E, Droste SK, Ohl F, Reul JMHM. Regular voluntary exercise reduces anxiety-related behaviour and impulsiveness in mice. Behav Brain Res 2004; 155:197-206.

[55]   Collins A, Hill LE, Chandramohan Y, Whitcomb D, Droste SK, Reul JMHM. Exercise improves cognitive responses to psychological stress through enhancement of epigenetic mechanisms and gene expression in the dentate gyrus. PLoS One 2009; 4:e4330.

[56]   Herman JP, Figueiredo H, Mueller NK, Ulrich-Lai Y, Ostrander MM, Choi DC *et al.* Central mechanisms of stress integration: hierarchical circuitry controlling hypothalamo-pituitary-adrenocortical responsiveness. Front Neuroendocrinol 2003; 24:151-180.

[57]   Treves A, Rolls ET. Computational analysis of the role of the hippocampus in memory. Hippocampus 1994; 4:374-391.

[58]   Rolls ET, Kesner RP. A computational theory of hippocampal function, and empirical tests of the theory. Prog Neurobiol 2006; 79:1-48

[59]   Papadopoulos A, Chandramohan Y, Collins A, Droste SK, Nutt DJ, Reul JMHM. GABAergic control of novelty stress-responsive epigenetic and gene expression mechanisms in the rat dentate gyrus. Eur Neuropsychopharmacol 2011; 21:316-324.

[60]   Hill LE, Droste SK, Nutt DJ, Linthorst AC, Reul JMHM. Voluntary exercise alters GABAA receptor subunit and glutamic acid decarboxylase-67 gene expression in the rat forebrain. J Psychopharmacol 2010; 24:745-756.

[61]   McGee SL, Fairlie E, Garnham AP, Hargreaves M. Exercise-induced histone modifications in human skeletal muscle. J Physiol 2009; 587:5951-5958.

[62]   Hargreaves DC, Horng T, Medzhitov R. Control of inducible gene expression by signal-dependent transcriptional elongation. Cell 2009; 138:129-145.

[63]   McKinsey TA, Zhang CL, Olson EN. Control of muscle development by dueling HATs and HDACs. Curr Opin Genet Dev 2001; 11:497-504.

[64]   Fischle W, Dequiedt F, Hendzel MJ, Guenther MG, Lazar MA, Voelter W *et al.* Enzymatic activity associated with class II HDACs is dependent on a multiprotein complex containing HDAC3 and SMRT/N-CoR. Mol Cell 2002; 9:45-57.

[65]   Ordovas JM, Mooser V. Nutrigenomics and nutrigenetics. Curr Opin Lipidol 2004; 15:101-108.

[66]   Bouchard L, Rabasa-Lhoret R, Faraj M, Lavoie ME, Mill J, Perusse L *et al.* Differential epigenomic and transcriptomic responses in subcutaneous adipose tissue between low and high responders to caloric restriction. Am J Clin Nutr 2010; 91:309-320.

[67]   Campion J, Milagro FI, Goyenechea E, Martinez JA. TNF-alpha promoter methylation as a predictive biomarker for weight-loss response. Obesity (Silver Spring) 2009; 17:1293-1297.

[68]   Milagro FI, Campion J, Cordero P, Goyenechea E, Gomez-Uriz AM, Abete I *et al.* A dual epigenomic approach for the search of obesity biomarkers: DNA methylation in relation to diet-induced weight loss. FASEB J 2011; 25:1378-1389.

[69]   Waterland RA, Travisano M, Tahiliani KG, Rached MT, Mirza S. Methyl donor supplementation prevents transgenerational amplification of obesity. Int J Obes (Lond) 2008; 32:1373-1379.

CHAPTER 4

Epigenetic Mechanisms in Drug Addiction and its Clinical Management

Carla Sanchis-Segura[*] and Marta Miquel

Psychobiology Section Universitat Jaume I, Castelló de la Plana, Spain

Abstract: There is increasing evidence that the environment modifies individual genotypes through epigenetic mechanisms, creating behavioral traits and leaving persistent memories of past events. In post-mitotic cells such as neurons, chromatin modifications provide not only transient but also stable (or even permanent) epigenetic marks. These could promote, maintain or block transcriptional processes that, in turn, participate in the molecular adaptations underlying behavioral changes. Accordingly, epigenetics has become a central topic in several domains of neuroscience, including neurobiological approaches to drug addiction. In this chapter we summarize current evidence for the involvement of epigenetic mechanisms in the promotion of drug consumption and addictive behavior. We also suggest how the same epigenetic mechanisms could be used to improve the clinical management of these disorders.

Keywords: Addiction, epigenetics, histone posttranslational modifications, DNA methylation, therapeutics.

4.1. FOREWORD

In this chapter we review the evidence implicating epigenetic mechanisms in drug consumption and addictive behavior. Further, we also suggest ways in which the same epigenetic mechanisms might be used to improve the clinical management of addiction. However, this chapter does not discuss how epigenetic mechanisms might mediate drug effects in organs or tissues other than the brain. Nor do we review current knowledge of how drugs of abuse might act as teratological agents, altering developmental processes or interrupting the homeostatic activity of somatic systems. Although all these aspects are relevant when considering how drugs of abuse interact with the genome through epigenetic mechanisms, a complete description and discussion of such interactions lies outside the scope of

---

[*]**Address correspondence to Carla Sanchis-Segura:** Psychobiology section, Universitat Jaume I, Avda. Sos Baynat S/N, 12071 Castelló de la Plana, Spain; Tel: 34-964 72 9933; Fax: 964729267; E-mail: csanchis@psb.uji.es

Marcelina Párrizas, Rosa Gasa and Perla Kaliman (Eds)

this chapter. Consequently, this chapter is limited to the discussion of the involvement of epigenetic mechanisms in drug consumption and addiction-related phenomena.

4.2. EPIGENETICS AND COMPLEX PHENOTYPES

All individuals of the same species share the same genes, but those that reproduce sexually acquire genetic distinctiveness from the unique combination of alleles they inherited from their parents. Equipped with different genotypes, individuals differ in their morphological, physiological and behavioral characteristics and, consequently, in their chances of survival. However, it would be a mistake to interpret this co-variation as causation, and conclude that genotypic differences determine phenotypic diversity. Thus, as it is clearly illustrated by animal clones and monozygotic twins (which are considered genetically identical individuals), phenotypic variation also occurs in the absence of genetic differences. This indicates that non-genomic (*i.e.* environmental) factors contribute significantly to the phenotype. The succession of environmental challenges further increases the discrepancies between genotype and phenotype. Even between genetically identical individuals, phenotypic variation tends to increase over time, despite the fact that the inherited genome remains virtually unchanged throughout life. Thus, the relationship between genotype and phenotype is complex, and it cannot be understood without considering the role of environmental factors.

The role of both genetic and environmental factors in determining phenotypes and susceptibility to disease is generally acknowledged, but often erroneously conceptualized. Both the constitutive characteristics and the development of an individual can only be understood as the result of an uninterrupted and constantly changing interaction between the individual's genome and its environment. Interaction is the key word, and it introduces implications other than addition. That is, genetic and environmental factors do not simply add their relative independent contribution. Indeed, beyond statistical effects, there is no such thing as a "relative independent contribution" of genetic or environmental factors. When applied to the study of any biological system (or individual behavior) notions such as a "gene main effect" or "environment main effect" become senseless. Furthermore, the concept of interaction implies that the influence of one factor (or set of factors) on a complex phenotype might change its magnitude, and even its direction, depending on the values of the other factors. Thus, for example, it has been shown that the contribution of a particular allele of the *rhMAOA-LPR* gene to aggressive behavior in rhesus monkeys depends on individual rearing conditions. The low-activity-associated allele is associated with greater aggression in mother-reared male monkeys, but less aggression in pair-reared [1, 2]. Similar gene-environment interactions have been reported as major determinants of other behavior patterns such as alcohol consumption [3] and they may occur throughout life. Thus, although they did not differ in their basal alcohol consumption, mice lacking a functional corticotropin-releasing hormone type 1 receptor (CRH1), but not their respective littermate controls, showed a life-long enhanced alcohol intake after stress exposure [4]. From these examples it is clear that phenotypic variation is the result of gene-environment interactions and that the contribution of genetic or environmental factors cannot be considered separately.

However, concluding that phenotypes arise from complex and non-additive interactions of genetic and environmental factors is not enough. In fact, this proposal becomes largely devoid of meaning and usefulness if it is not accompanied by the development of a unitary theoretical framework to describe the interplay between both kinds of factors in biologically relevant terms. Epigenetics is a scientific approach that allows the construction of such a conceptual framework. Increasingly, it also provides suitable technology to explore and modify gene-environment interactions. More specifically, epigenetics deals with cellular mechanisms that control reversible gene expression states. Such mechanisms may be inheritable, but they do not involve alterations to the DNA sequence.

By controlling gene expression, epigenetic mechanisms promote and maintain cell lineage, and also facilitate cellular plasticity. During development, stem cells differentiate into a wide array of specialized cell types that function as part of a biological system. This differentiation process and the maintenance of the cell lineage are ensured by epigenetic mechanisms [5]. In postmitotic cells, by favoring or reducing the access of regulatory proteins to DNA, epigenetic mechanisms govern the metabolic status of the cell and protect its homeostasis in a changing environment [6]. Likewise, any need or extracellular insult can only be met through selective gene expression, which provides (and limits) the molecular elements needed to restore homeostasis. Therefore, cells provide the context for a continuous dialog between the genome and non-genetic factors, which maintains, updates or redefines the cellular phenotype. Because most of the cellular elements involved in this interactive process are subjected to extracellular regulation, this dialog participates in those occurring at higher levels (organs and systems). Simultaneously, the cellular phenotype (derived from environmentally reversible gene expression states) dictates the potential role and current activity of the cell within its corresponding organ and system, thus finally contributing to the individual's behavior and its interaction with macro-environmental factors (Fig. **1**).

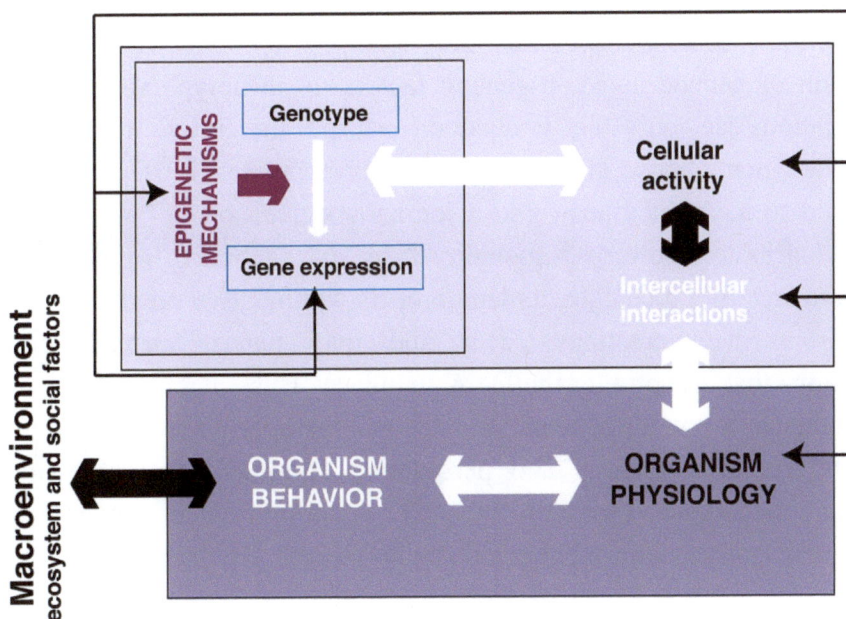

Figure 1: Modular conceptualization of environmental factors and their interactions with the inherited genotype. The activity of cells, physiological systems and organisms are understood to be the result of an uninterrupted and continuous interaction between genetic and non-genetic (*i.e.* environmental) factors.

In this regard, epigenetic mechanisms not only regulate gene expression by enhancing or preventing the DNA-protein interactions required for transcription, but they also provide a system by which states of gene expression can be "memorized". In contrast to histone acetylation, which is rather labile, DNA methylation and perhaps other epigenetic marks may provide the anchoring points for more stable, if not permanent, gene expression networks. This additional layer of information stored at the chromatin level becomes the source of inter-individual-epigenetic and, consequently, phenotypic variation. Thus, the patterns of epigenetic modification in monozygotic twin pairs diverge as they become older, especially if they have different life styles regarding nutrition, physical activity or drug consumption [7]. Accordingly, how environmental stimuli and events shape the "epigenetic landscape" defining the individual's traits (and its proneness to diseases) within the span of one lifetime, and perhaps even across generations, has become an area of major research interest [8-10].

In summary, it is neither possible nor useful to try to separate the relative contribution of genetic and non-genetic factors to phenotype variation. Indeed, such variation can only be understood as the integrative result of gene-environment interactions. This was beautifully expressed by Donald O. Hebb, who is said to have once answered a journalist's question of "which, nature or nurture, contributes more to personality?" by asking back: "which contributes more to the area of a rectangle, its length or its width?". We now know that such gene-environment interactions occur and may persist through chromatin modifications that do not alter the DNA sequence. This epigenetic level provides the mechanisms to "write", "read" and "erase" the appropriate chromatin marks and, therefore, to transiently and persistently regulate gene expression, thus promoting phenotypic variation as well as allowing the organization of appropriate responses to environmental challenges and events.

4.3. ADDICTION AS A NEUROPLASTICITY DISORDER: INVOLVEMENT OF EPIGENETIC MECHANISMS

Neurons, as postmitotic mature nerve cells, have highly specialized functions that collectively determine our perception and responses to external stimuli, but also our ability to store such events as memories. The vast number of nerve cells (and their interconnections) and their extraordinary adaptive capacity allow the central nervous system (CNS) to carry out those higher-order functions in response to environmental demands. Neuroplasticity is the brain's ability to adapt to change.

Although neuroplastic changes are triggered in response to multiple external stimuli and their consequences are reflected at several levels (behavioral, anatomical, electrical, synaptic, *etc.*), long-term plasticity is always made possible through changes in gene expression [11]. In the single neuron, these phenomena are derived from the dynamic (and probably epigenetically regulated) pattern of gene expression, which determines both its transient and its long-lasting responses [6, 12].

Plastic changes in nerve cells underlie all types of memory formation [13] and allow neurons to respond appropriately to biologically relevant stimuli. Plasticity occurs in motivation and learning/memory-related neural circuits, so individuals can seek out and remember stimuli that are advantageous to survival, and avoid potential dangers. Neuroplasticity also underlies pathological or non-adaptive processes triggered by environmental stimuli. Thus, emotional or physical stress results in persistent functional and structural changes in different brain circuits, which can lead to anxiety and mood disorders [14]. Some of these changes are reversed by behavioral and pharmacological interventions and might reflect the brain's ability to generate new forms of plasticity. Similarly, behavioral changes observed after chronic exposure to drugs of abuse, such as tolerance, dependence and addictive behavior appear or are maintained long after the drugs have been cleared from the organism, and they cannot be attributed to acute effects of the interaction of the drugs with their primary molecular targets. These disorders arise from the wide array of structural and functional neuroplastic processes induced by the drug [11, 15].

Drugs of abuse such as cocaine, morphine, ethanol or nicotine modify the structure and activity of several brain systems, including those governing motivational and learning/memory processes. Thus, for example, morphine and cocaine alter the density of dendritic spines on medium spiny neurons in the Nucleus Accumbens (NAcc), especially in animals self-administering the drug [16]. Other drug-induced changes in neuron morphology have been described in the ventral tegmental area [17, 18]. Drugs of abuse also induce changes in glutamatergic synaptic strength. These can be long lasting, depending on several factors including whether the drugs are received passively or actively self-administered [19]. Further research is needed to elucidate how these and other drug-induced structural and functional changes relate to specific behavioral phenomena [20]. However, it is generally acknowledged that the neuroplastic changes induced by drugs of abuse have a wide range of effects. They alter how a person perceives motivationally relevant stimuli, they establish new behavioral repertoires and habits, and they precipitate the progressive loss of control over behavior that typifies addictive behavior [15, 21-23]. Drugs of abuse not only generate powerful memories and behavioral habits, but they also inhibit further induction of synaptic plasticity in neural systems involved in motivational and learning-memory processes [16, 24, 25], perhaps accounting for the addict's reduced ability to acquire new behavioral strategies that might compete with drug-seeking behavior [15]. Not surprisingly, addiction has been described as a "learning and memory disorder" [26], a "motivational disorder" [27] and a "neuroplasticity disorder" [15] characterized by compulsive drug-seeking/taking behavior.

In addition to the neuroplastic changes underlying the maintenance of drug seeking/taking behavior, drugs of abuse promote other forms of plasticity in the neural and non-neural cell populations directly affected by the drugs. These homeostatic cellular adaptations are responsible for the development of clinically relevant phenomena, such as tolerance and dependence. Although these conditions were once recognized as important signs of addiction (a viewpoint that still remains in some psychiatric diagnostic manuals; *e.g.* DSM-IV) it is now recognized that they are neither necessary nor sufficient for a person to be considered an addict [28]. Both phenomena without compulsive drug seeking/taking behavior are commonly observed in patients that are subjected to non-voluntary long-term to chronic treatment with opiates [29] or benzodiazepines [30]. On the other hand, compulsive use and multiple relapses can be observed in cocaine-, nicotine-, or amphetamine-addicted users who have not experienced strong withdrawal symptoms. Remarkably, in contrast to the neuroplastic changes underlying the maintenance of drug seeking/taking behavior, the ability of drugs to promote the homeostatic cellular adaptations leading to tolerance and dependence varies widely. It depends on the expression patterns of each drug's receptors and the intracellular signaling mechanisms engaged in each case [26]. Moreover, the cellular plastic processes associated with tolerance or dependence are shorter-lived than those produced in cells of the neural systems governing motivational and learning-memory processes. In consequence, relapse rather than drug detoxification is seen as the major problem in the clinical management of addicted patients [31].

In summary, after chronic exposure, drugs of abuse produce a wide array of neural changes. From a functional perspective, these changes can be classified in two main categories: homeostatic adaptations, which can be defined as negative feedback responses, and non-homeostatic adaptations, which underlie long-lasting positive feedback responses to drugs and drug-related stimuli. These two types of drug-induced change are clearly dissociable regarding their behavioral consequences as well as their molecular and neuroanatomical determinants but, like all forms of long-lasting neuroplasticity, they finally depend on differently regulated gene expression patterns. Not surprisingly, over the last two decades a substantial amount of research in the drug-addiction field has been devoted to the exploration of drug-induced changes in gene expression [11, 15, 32].

However, although activation of several intracellular signaling pathways and transcription factors has been described in response to drug exposure, little is known about the mechanisms by which chronic drug exposure persistently alters the expression of specific genes. Accumulating evidence indicates that drug-induced chromatin modifications may contribute to the maintenance of long-lasting changes in gene expression and ultimately to the development/maintenance of addictive behavior. Although preliminary, this knowledge may also provide a new basis for the treatment and clinical management of addiction.

4.4. CHROMATIN   MODIFICATIONS   AND   DRUG-INDUCED BEHAVIORAL EFFECTS

As mentioned above, it is generally assumed that the development and maintenance of addictive behavior, as well as other clinically relevant phenomena derived from chronic drug exposure (*e.g.* physical dependence), mainly arise from the ability of drugs to trigger multiple structural and functional CNS modifications that outlive the drug's availability in the organism. These changes (usually referred to as "drug-induced neuroplasticity") seem to be supported by similar mechanisms to those previously identified as underlying different kinds of learning and memory or triggered in response to other environmental challenges (*e.g.* stress), and inevitably require changes in gene expression [11]. Accordingly, how these drugs trigger changes in gene expression in neurons has become a major focus of interest in the elucidation of the brain mechanisms supporting drug consumption and, in some individuals, the transition to addiction. Over the last 5 years interest has focused on the possible role of epigenetic mechanisms in gene expression in drug-induced neuroplasticity, and these studies will be summarized here.

The appeal of epigenetic mechanisms in the drug addiction field (as in many other topics within neurobiology) arises from the belief that chromatin modifications could lead to stable gene expression patterns in postmitotic neurons and, consequently to behavioral regularities. Fast growing evidence supports the notion that drugs of abuse trigger post-translational modifications of histones, such as acetylation, phosphorylation and methylation, as well as DNA methylation. These modifications can promote changes in gene expression and behavior. The involvement of specific epigenetic mechanisms and their functional significance may vary according to the duration (acute *vs.* chronic) of drug exposure and many other factors. Thus, since this quest has only just started and initial studies have merely provided a "proof of concept" rather than systematic information, the data available on the involvement of epigenetic mechanisms in drug consumption/addiction are necessarily scattered. We still lack a comprehensive picture of how epigenetic mechanisms might be relevant in drug consumption, or addiction, or their treatment.

On the following pages we review the evidence for the involvement of epigenetic mechanisms in drug-induced neuroplastic and behavioral changes. For organizational purposes, the roles of specific epigenetic mechanisms in drug effects are discussed separately. Because these epigenetic mechanisms have been dealt with in Chapter 1, their general principles are not introduced. Similarly, details on behavioral tests and their significance for drug consumption/addiction will also be omitted. If needed, this information can easily be found elsewhere [33, 34].

4.4.1. Histone Post-Translational Modifications

As mentioned above, the study of the involvement of epigenetic mechanisms in drug consumption/addiction is very recent. At first [35, 36], as in research in the learning/memory field, interest was focused on histone post-translational modifications. Of these, histone acetylation and phosphorylation received the most attention. Thus, these two kinds of histone post-translational modification, together with recent evidence on the role of histone methylation in drug neuroplasticity and behavior, will be reviewed below. Conversely, histone sumoylation, deimination or ubiquitylation, and a possible role of the replacement of histone variants in the neurobiological mechanisms governing drug abuse and addictive behavior remain unexplored and they will not be further commented here.

4.4.1.1. Histone Methylation

Histone methylation is particularly complex, as each possible methylation site can exist in mono-, di- and trimethylated states, each one recruiting specific enzymes and cofactors with a wide range of effects on transcriptional activity. Further, each of these methylation states can induce opposite effects on gene expression, depending on the specific lysine that is methylated. Besides, histone methylation often occurs in combination with other post-translational modifications, such as histone acetylation and phosphorylation, and it may also interact with DNA methylation. The study of the involvement of histone methylation in drug-induced neuroplasticity and behavior is only recent [37, 38], but it is likely to be an area of immediate growth, particularly because of its possible scaffolding role for DNA methylation [39, 40].

Although repeated psychostimulant exposure mainly results in gene activation in the NAcc [41], the complex transcriptome triggered by this treatment also requires the active suppression of particular genes. Thus, using a ChIP-on-chip based approach, Renthal *et al.* (2009) showed that chronic cocaine administration increases H3 and H4 acetylation marks (previously linked to gene activation) as well as dimethylation of H3 at lysines 9 (H3K9) and 27 (H3K27) (which are involved in gene suppression) [38]. In this study, 898 gene promoters exhibited enhanced H3K9 and H3K27 dimethylation as compared to the 1004 and 692 gene promoters that displayed increased H3 and H4 acetylation, respectively. Conversely, 80 and 120 genes showed reduced H3 and H4 acetylation respectively, but co-occurrence of reduced H3/H4 acetylation and increased H3K9/H3K27 dimethylation was minimal and only found in 2% of the gene promoters evaluated.

Renthal *et al.* (2009) also identified a cohort of genes displaying reduced histone acetylation and methylation after chronic cocaine exposure [38]. A similar reduction of H3K9 dimethylation after repeated cocaine administration was also reported in a more recent study [42]. In this later study, H3K27 dimethylation was slightly, but not significantly, reduced, leading to a global decrease (rather than an increase, as in the case of the study by Renthal *et al.* 2009 [38]) of euchromatic H3 dimethylated levels, which was accompanied by an increase in gene expression. Therefore, although some particular aspects of those two studies seem difficult to reconcile at present, they both suggest that cocaine may enhance the expression of at least some genes by reducing histone methylation processes at their promoters.

The reduction of H3K9 dimethylation observed by Maze *et al.* (2010) after repeated cocaine administration was derived from the down-regulation of two lysine methylases that specifically catalyze this reaction: G9a and GLP [42]. G9a might be especially interesting in regard to long-term neuroplasticity because, besides its role in histone methylation, it seems to facilitate the recruitment of other enzymes involved in DNA methylation [40]. Interestingly, G9a (but not GLP) regulates dendritic plasticity in the NAcc as well as cocaine-induced conditioned place preference (CPP). More specifically, repeated cocaine administration decreased G9a binding and H3K9 dimethylation levels at the promoters of genes such as *Arc* (*activity-regulated cytoskeleton-associated protein*) and *Bdnf* (*brain-derived neurotrophic factor*), thus resulting in increased spine formation in this brain area as well as CPP. Both sets of cocaine effects were increased after inducing selective downregulation of G9a expression by the delivery of appropriate viral vectors expressing the recombinase Cre in the NAcc of adult G9a$^{fl/fl}$ mice. Conversely, overexpression of G9a blocked CPP as well as the development of cocaine-induced dendritic morphological changes in cocaine-treated animals. Taken together, these data indicate that reduced G9a-mediated

H3K9 dimethylation at the promoters of several genes is crucial to the ability of repeated cocaine administration to promote structural forms of plasticity at the dendrites of NAcc neurons as well as behavioral effects such as CPP.

These findings have been linked to Delta FosB (DFosB), which is one of the transcription factors most widely studied in drug-induced neuroplasticity [43, 44]. Evidence reported by Maze *et al.* (2010) indicates that G9a is recruited to the *FosB* promoter and limits DFosB induction in response to initial cocaine administration [42]. However, conversely to the rest of Fos family proteins, DFosB is resistant to proteosomal degradation and, as drug exposure is repeated, it accumulates in the NAcc neurons [43, 44]. DFosB persists long (1-2 months) after psychostimulant exposure is ceased, and acts as either an activator or a repressor of gene expression depending on the target gene [43], probably through recruitment of specific epigenetic machinery [37, 38, 44]. Interestingly, DFosB overexpression, which results in enhanced cocaine-induced CPP and locomotor sensitization [45], may also promote *G9a* (but not *GLP*) repression, leading to a reduction of H3K9 dimethylation at several genes targeted by this histone methyltransferase. This not only mimicks cocaine-induced dendritic neuroplastic changes but also triggers a positive feedback loop that might boost its own expression [42].

In summary, although the study of histone methylation is relatively new, there is convincing evidence for the involvement of this epigenetic mechanism in drug-induced neuroplasticity as well as behavior. However, chronic exposure to psychostimulants can either increase or decrease histone methylation at specific gene promoters, raising the concern that global measurements of post-translational histone modifications might be poorly informative about their functional consequences. On the other hand, although histone methylation can be considered as relatively short-lived, it might facilitate DNA methylation [40]. Current evidence has already linked this epigenetic mechanism to at least some forms of drug-induced structural neuroplasticity as well as their long-lasting behavioral consequences.

4.4.1.2. Histone Phosphorylation

Histone phosphorylation is generally associated with transcriptional activation; it can be observed on the promoters of immediate early genes such as *c-fos* when they are induced by cAMP or by glutamate treatment in cultured striatal neurons [46]. The most widely studied histone phosphorylation site is serine 10 on histone H3 (H3S10). The histone acetylase enzyme Gcn5 is recruited to gene promoters bearing H3S10 phosphorylation marks. As a result, the neighboring lysine (H3K9) is often acetylated (phospho-acetylation), thus reducing the likelihood of a possible (repressive) H3K9 methylation [47]. Accordingly, phospho-acetylation seems to accompany highly activated gene states and is activated in response to drugs of abuse [35, 48-50].

Cocaine [35, 49, 51] or morphine [50] administration increases histone H3S10 phosphorylation in the striatum. This effect was not observed after acute ethanol administration [50], a finding that contrasts with the ability of alcohol and its metabolites to promote histone H3S10 and H3S28 phosphorylation in cultured hepatocytes [52].

The ability of psychostimulants to increase histone H3S10 phosphorylation is readily observable in both bulk histone phosphorylation levels as well as at the promoters of specific genes such as *c-fos* and *c-Jun* [53]. Several protein kinase families including ribosomal subunit protein S6 kinases (RSKs) and mitogen and stress activated protein kinases (MSKs) might mediate these events [48]. Additionally, cocaine-induced Protein Phosphatase-2A (PP2A)-mediated dephosphorylation of the dopamine- and cAMP-regulated phosphoprotein of 32 kDa (DARPP-32) promotes nuclear accumulation of this protein, which through its inhibitory activity over Protein Phosphatase 1 (PP1) increases H3S10 phosphorylation [51]. Interestingly, at the striatal level, the increase in histone H3 phosphorylation triggered by cocaine is restricted to neurons expressing the dopamine receptor D1, whereas the dopamine receptor D2 antagonist haloperidol produces the same effect but only in D2-expressing neurons [54].

As indicated above, H3S10 phosphorylation is often accompanied by the acetylation of some lysines (K9, K14) in the same histone tail. Initially, it was believed that both histone modifications played a sequential role (H3S10 phosphorylation facilitating K14 acetylation) in the nucleosomal remodeling processes that allows the incorporation of transcription factors and, consequently, gene expression. However, it has now been established that both post-translational modifications operate "in parallel" when promoting nucleosomal remodeling processes at specific gene loci [48]. Indeed, in response to acute cocaine or morphine administration, selective increases of H3S10 phosphorylation in the absence of acetylation changes in this histone have been reported [35, 50].

To our knowledge, no author has addressed the role of histone phosphorylation or phospho-acetylation in the behavioral effects derived from acute or chronic drug exposure. Nevertheless, several studies have shown that some of the protein kinases and phosphatases that could mediate H3S10 phosphorylation (and many other substrates) are also involved in some of the behavioral consequences observed after chronic drug administration. Thus, MSK1 knockout mice show delayed locomotor sensitization in response to cocaine [49], whereas knock-in mice bearing a point mutation critical for PP2A-mediated dephosphorylation of DARP32 (S97A-DARP-32 mice) display not only reduced H3S10 phosphorylation but also reduced cocaine-induced CPP and cocaine- and morphine-induced locomotor sensitization [51].

4.4.1.3. Histone Acetylation

Histone acetylation is promoted by acetyltransferase enzymes (HATs) and reduced by the activity of histone deacetylases (HDACs). Acetylation occurs on histones H2A, H2B, H3, and H4. However, in the context of drug addiction, research on this epigenetic modification has mainly focused on H3, where it can occur on the N-terminal tails at lysines 9, 14, 18, and 23, and on H4 at lysines 5, 8, 12, and 16. In general, histone acetylation is considered an "activating epigenetic mark". Thus, histone acetylation is believed to upregulate gene expression by two main mechanisms. First, acetylation of lysine residues reduces their positive charge and consequently their electrostatic attraction to the negatively-charged backbone of DNA, thus promoting the "relaxed" chromatin structure required to allow the access of transcription factors to the appropriate underlying DNA sequences. Second, acetylated histones serve as docking sites that would facilitate the binding of proteins containing bromodomains.

Studies assessing the ability of drugs of abuse to increase bulk histone acetylation in the CNS have provided conflicting results. Thus, acute administration of cocaine promotes an increase of histone H4 acetylation in the striatum [49].

However, other authors did not observe such an increase in response to cocaine, morphine or ethanol [50, 55]. Similarly, increases [56, 57], decreases [58] or no change [50] in bulk histone acetylation levels in response to chronic drug exposure have been reported.

This disparity might be due, at least in part, to the diversity in the treatment conditions (*i.e.* drug used and dosage), subject characteristics and the brain regions analyzed. Indeed, as illustrated by Pascual *et al.* (2009), the same drug treatment produces a different outcome depending on the subjects' age (young rats are more prone to exhibit histone acetylation changes) [59]. Moreover, even in the same subject, the same treatment might promote opposite changes in different brain areas (increases of H3 and H4 histone acetylation in the prefrontal cortex and NAcc, but decreases in other regions of the striatum). However, as mentioned for histone methylation, these results also reveal that raw measures of global histone acetylation do not capture the complex and specific pattern of histone modifications triggered by drugs of abuse in specific DNA regions. Indeed, if histone acetylation changes regulate gene expression, these changes should not occur in the whole genome of heterogeneous neuronal populations belonging to large anatomical brain structures (*i.e.* striatum) but rather at the promoters of restricted groups of genes of particular cell populations. Thus, although the administration of drugs of abuse might result in global changes of histone acetylation levels, these are actually due to altered acetylation at a restricted number of specific genes. However, neither the identity of the genes that are subjected to acetylation/deacetylation processes nor the consequences for their expression rate can be derived from global measurements. In consequence, global measures of histone acetylation should not be used to justify any conclusions about the functional consequences of acetylation-related processes for drug-induced neuroplasticity or behavior. More likely, they will be progressively abandoned and replaced by more specific approaches.

Acute and chronic administration of drugs of abuse as well as drug abstinence promote different forms of neuroplasticity that lead to different clinically relevant phenomena [15]. In recent years, some of these forms of drug-related neuroplasticity have been linked to acetylation/deacetylation processes at different histones of the promoters of specific genes [60]. Thus, acute administration of cocaine transiently increases the acetylation levels of histone H4 at specific loci of genes such as *c-fos and Fosb*, as well as their expression [35, 49]. This increase in histone H4 acetylation was not observed in the loci of other genes such as *Tubb* (*beta tubulin*), whose expression remained unaltered after drug exposure. On the contrary, as drug administration is repeated, these epigenetic modifications change dramatically and point to a prominent albeit unexplained role of acetylation/deacetylation processes at H3 rather than H4). Furthermore, genes that exhibited similar epigenetic modifications after acute drug administration can undergo disparate regulatory processes as drug exposure is extended. Thus, *c-fos* expression desensitizes in response to chronic psychostimulant administration, and this progressive reduction of its transcriptional activity is associated with the normalization of histone acetylation levels at the gene promoter [35, 61]. Conversely, histone H3 acetylation at the *FosB* promoter was increased in response to the same cocaine treatment. Such an increase in acetylation at H3, but not H4, in response to chronic cocaine administration is also found at the promoters of other genes, such as *Npy* (*neuropeptide Y*) [62], *Cdk5* (*cyclin-dependent kinase 5*) and *Bdnf* [35]. These promoters show a further increase in both H3 acetylation and transcriptional activity after the end of drug exposure. Similarly, the reduction of *Egr-1* expression during cocaine abstinence is accompanied by a decrease in histone H3 acetylation at its promoter [62].

If these studies have shown that drugs of abuse alter chromatin structure at specific genes, genome-wide studies of histone acetylation might provide a more general view of the genes that show activating/repressing marks after drug exposure. They may also disclose unexpected targets and signaling pathways to be further explored. In this regard, a study using a ChIP-on-chip approach [38] revealed that after repeated cocaine administration the promoters of 1004 and 692 genes of NAcc cells are hyperacetylated at H3 or H4, respectively. Several genes (*e.g. Arc, Cart* (*cocaine- and amphetamine-regulated transcript*), *Cdk5*, or *Per1* (*period homolog 1*)) that increase their expression in response to drug exposure fell within this group, whereas genes usually down-regulated by the same treatments (*e.g. Mtap2* (*microtubule-associated protein 2*)) appeared among the 83 and 123 genes exhibiting hypoacetylated levels at either H3 or H4. In most cases, acetylation levels were maximal in a specific and relatively narrow region (between -500 and +200 bp) situated at transcription start sites, although significant variation in the acetylation patterns of different genes was observed. Surprisingly, only 15% of regulated gene promoters showed concurrent hyperacetylation of H3 and H4, whereas simultaneous H3 and H4 hypoacetylation was only observed in 1% of cases. Finally, some genes known to be involved in drug-induced neuroplasticity and behavior such as *Mef2* (*myocyte enhancer factor 2*) or *Hdac4* (*histone deacetylase 4*) do not seem to change their expression despite bearing histone acetylation marks at their promoters. However, the expression of these genes might be modified later, as has been described for other addiction-relevant genes such as *Bdnf* [35]. In summary, these results, together with those mentioned above in relation to the low co-occurrence of acetylation and methylation-related marks (see section 4.4.1.1), demonstrate that repeated cocaine administration activates several largely independent epigenetic mechanisms. In contrast, a single kind of epigenetic modification located at a single histone type might promote changes in the expression of a vast set of genes that can endure or even begin after the cessation of drug administration [38].

Little is known about the exact molecular mechanisms through which drugs of abuse produce these local changes in histone acetylation, although the scattered evidence available suggests that multiple enzymatic pathways and mechanisms might be involved. Thus, for example, acute alcohol administration reduces HDAC activity while increasing expression of CBP (a protein with HAT activity) in the medial amygdala regions [56]. This extends previous reports on the ethanol-enhancing effects of proteins displaying HAT activity in other tissues (*e.g.* liver [63]). The acetylating actions of CBP have also been associated with the hyperacetylation at the *FosB* gene promoter observed after cocaine administration [36]. On the other hand, although it does not necessarily modify their expression levels ([35], but see also [64]), chronic psychostimulant administration seems to alter the activity of several type I/II HDACs by multiple indirect mechanisms. Thus, *via* a mechanism that probably involves different Ca2+/calmodulin-dependent kinases [65], chronic cocaine administration is associated with increased HDAC5 phosphorylation in the NAcc [66], which facilitates its nuclear export and reduces its repression of gene expression. Similarly, repeated amphetamine administration leads to the dissociation of the CREB:HDAC1 complex, thereby facilitating histone acetylation and CREB phosphorylation. The mechanism probably involves PP1, which is also attached to this complex [57]. Conversely, HDAC1 seems to be recruited by DFosB to promote the progressive desensitization of *c-fos* expression observed in response to a similar drug treatment [61].

Drug-induced histone acetylation/deacetylation and its effects on gene expression might have a significant role in drug abuse and the development and maintenance of drug seeking/taking behavior. Initial evidence has been provided by studies involving the administration of inhibitors of type I/II HDACs (hereafter termed HDACi). These studies have shown that several behavioral effects induced by a wide range of drugs of abuse are boosted when histone deacetylation is reduced. Thus, the administration of the HDACi sodium butyrate increases cocaine self-administration ([67-69]). Further, systemic administration of sodium butyrate and other HDACi also enhances the ability of cocaine [35, 66, 70, 71] and morphine [50], but apparently not nicotine [72], to produce CPP. Accordingly the administration of HAT inhibitors might reduce drug-induced CPP [71]. These results implicate histone acetylation in the neuroplasticity processes underlying the ability of drugs to set up and support approach behavior towards drug cues (a form of drug seeking behavior measurable in CPP procedures) as well as drug-taking behavior.

This conclusion has been further supported, but also refined, by experiments involving genetic manipulation of specific HDACs. Thus, overexpression of HDAC4 or HDAC5 (but not HDAC9) in the NAcc results in a reduction of cocaine-induced CPP [66] and self-administration [68]. This finding, coupled with the observation that chronic, but not acute, cocaine exposure induces HDAC5 phosphorylation and its nuclear export, provides a putative mechanism by which the expression of HDAC5 target genes and the behavioral responses to this drug could be progressively enhanced [37]. Experimental evidence consistent with this proposal has been provided in HDAC5 knockout mice, which show enhanced responses to chronic, but not acute, cocaine administration [66]. Similarly, selective deletion of Ca2+/calmodulin-dependent kinase IV (CaMKIV) in the striatum resulted in increased HDAC4 phosphorylation in the striatum as well as enhanced CPP after cocaine administration [73]. Although the exact mechanisms underlying this phenotype remain to be clarified, it is plausible that CamMKIV deletion could have led to the upregulation of other CaMKs, which could be responsible for the observed increased phosphorylation of HDAC4 and the enhanced response of this strain of mice to repeated cocaine administration.

Similarly, the progressive enhancement of locomotion (locomotor sensitization) resulting from repeated amphetamine, cocaine, ethanol or morphine administration is also boosted by the co-administration of HDACi [50, 57, 74]. A similar enhancement of locomotor sensitization was observed in mice displaying enhanced HDAC4 phosphorylation after CaMKIV deletion [73], whereas it was severely reduced in mice lacking an allele of CBP, a histone acetylating protein [36]. Once again, these results argue for an important role of histone acetylation/deacetylation in drug-induced neuroplasticity and its behavioral consequences. Indeed, as seen in experiments involving transient HDAC5 overexpression in the NAcc by means of HSV vectors [50, 66], mice treated with sodium butyrate during the development of morphine-induced sensitization also showed greater locomotion in a sensitization-expression test conducted seven days later. Therefore, similarly to the transient role proposed for CBP-HAT activity in long-term memory [75], it seems that HDACs exert a modulatory role during the induction of drug-induced neuroplasticity and that once these neural modifications have been established, their consequences remain and the participation of the HDACs may be dispensable. Accordingly, in several of those studies [36, 50, 57, 76] the effects of HDAC or HAT activity reduction on the development of drug-induced sensitization were paralleled by similar enhancing/reducing effects in the ability of these drugs to enhance the transcriptional activity of several genes implicated in the development of addictive behavior, such as *FosB* [43, 77] or *Per1* [78, 79]. As in the behavioral studies, the ability of morphine to enhance gene expression in sodium butyrate pre-treated mice was maintained when mice were re-challenged with morphine seven days after their last sodium butyrate injection [50].

Initial evidence suggests that histone acetylation may not be equally involved in all behavioral manifestations arising from drug-induced neuroplasticity. Thus, a recent study [50] has shown that the development of tolerance to the analgesic effects of morphine or to the motor-impairing effects of ethanol in mice is not affected by the co-administration of sodium butyrate. Similarly, co-administration of this HDACi with morphine or ethanol administration schedules that result in physical dependence does not modify the behavioral manifestations of the ethanol or morphine withdrawal syndrome [50]. However, the administration of another HDACi, trichostatin A, twenty-two hours after the termination of chronic forced alcohol consumption reduced anxiety-like behavior in alcohol-withdrawn rats [56]. These results suggest that the expression of withdrawal symptoms, but not the induction of physical dependence, might be modified by HDACi.

Thus, although much research is still needed, evidence indicates a much less important role of histone acetylation in the development of tolerance and dependence than in other behavioral consequences of chronic drug administration, such as CPP or locomotor sensitization. As mentioned above (section 4.3), although all these phenomena require changes in gene expression, tolerance and dependence rely on relatively short-lived homeostatic neuroplastic adaptations, *i.e.* negative feed-back mechanisms triggered after intense drug activation in the neural circuits directly activated by each drug. Accordingly, the likelihood and behavioral manifestation of these neuroadaptive processes is very different among drugs of different pharmacological families. Conversely, CPP and locomotor sensitization are useful behavioral tests to elucidate the neural mechanisms underlying some aspects of drug-seeking behavior (*i.e.* the Pavlovian approach) and incentive motivation [34]. These phenomena are considered key elements of addictive behavior [21, 22, 26, 79] and depend on non-homeostatic, long-lasting neural changes in the midbrain dopamine neurons and in several neural circuits that receive their input. Therefore, the evidence reviewed above opens the intriguing possibility that histone acetylation could be engaged in those long-lasting neuroplastic changes underlying the development and maintenance of addictive behavior, but not (or only to a lesser extent) in other (short-lived) neural adaptations triggered by drugs of abuse. Alternatively, the mechanisms underlying tolerance and dependence might admit less modulation, or the usually high drug doses required to induce those phenomena may contribute to masking a possible boosting effect of HDACi administration. Partial support for this proposal is provided by a study showing that sodium butyrate-fed flies exhibit a "tolerant-like" phenotype towards benzyl alcohol-induced sedation that is not further increased after a second intoxication episode [80]. However, the lack of effects of sodium butyrate on the development of tolerance to the motor incoordinating effects of alcohol and to the analgesic properties of morphine reported by Sanchis-Segura *et al.* (2009) were observed in experiments involving drug dosages equal to or lower than those at which this HDACi enhanced drug-induced locomotor sensitization and CPP [50]. Future studies may reveal whether the different temporal persistence and other differential characteristics of homeostatic and non-homeostatic forms of neuroplasticity triggered by drugs of abuse are related to a differential involvement of histone acetylation or other epigenetic mechanisms.

Another word of caution should be also introduced when trying to interpret the role of HAT and HDAC inhibitors in drug-induced neuroplasticity and behavioral effects. Thus, it is important to take into account that HATs and HDACs are actually lysine acetylases/deacetylases that shuttle between the nucleus and the cytoplasm, interacting with a large number of substrates. Indeed, reversible modification of lysine affects mRNA stability, and the localization, interaction, degradation and function of a large number of proteins. Hence, acetylation might be considered an intracellular signaling pathway that is almost as general as phosphorylation. The list of proteins activated/deactivated in response to acetylation includes several transcription factors (*e.g.* p53, YY1 or NF-kB), nuclear receptors (including Estrogen receptor a, Androgen receptor and SHP), chaperones (such as HSP90) as well as cytoskeleton/transport proteins (*e.g.* alpha-tubulin) and probably others (for a more extensive discussion of this topic see [81, 82]). Thus, even without considering a possible lack of specificity of HAT/HDAC inhibitors (*i.e.* effects in proteins other than those enzymes themselves), the administration of these compounds may affect a wide variety of cellular processes that cannot be easily dissociated. Consequently, finding an effect of the administration HAT/HDAC inhibitors on drug-induced neuroplasticity and behavior does not necessarily imply that this effect occurs at the epigenetic level or that it only depends on this kind of mechanism.

Indeed, the involvement of both epigenetic and non-epigenetic mechanisms in the ability of HDACi to modify at least some drug-induced behavioral effects has already been proposed [38, 50, 60]. In the study by Sanchis-Segura *et al.* (2009) the results of a detailed linear regression-based analysis of the effects of sodium butyrate on morphine-induced locomotor sensitization suggested that this HDACi might boost this behavioral effect by two separate mechanisms [50]. On the one hand, the almost instantaneous ability of sodium butyrate to enhance the increase in mouse locomotion observed after morphine administration might be more compatible with synaptic rather than genomic actions of this compound. On the other hand, the fact that sodium butyrate also increases the rate at which locomotion progressively increases with each repeated morphine injection (sensitization) seems more compatible with the development of long-lasting forms of plasticity that require gene expression changes and that might be regulated at the epigenetic level. More direct evidence for the involvement of non-genomic regulatory actions of HDACs has been provided by studying the sirtuin family of class III NAD-dependent deacetylases. In this regard, it has been reported that, conversely to the inhibition of other HDACs, a pharmacological reduction of sirtuin activity leads to a reduction of some behavioral effects of cocaine such as CPP, which seem to be due to the ability of sirtuins to regulate ERK phosphorylation, and hence the electrical excitability of NAcc medium spiny neurons, rather than to their histone deacetylating actions [38]. Therefore, although the levels of class III HDACs Sirt1 and Sirt2 in the NAcc are subjected to epigenetic regulation (*e.g.* repeated cocaine administration increase H3 acetylation at the promoters of the *Sirt1* and *Sirt 2* genes that leads to an enhancement of their expression levels through mechanisms probably involving DfosB recruitment, [38]), their actions on drug-induced neuroplasticity and behavior do not necessarily occur at this level.

In summary, histone acetylation is the most widely studied epigenetic mechanism in the context of drug abuse research. In this regard, it has been established that both acute and chronic drug administration enhance histone acetylation at the promoters of certain genes. Further, although conflicting results have been reported, it has been shown that pharmacological or genetic manipulation of the histone acetylating/deacetylating enzymes modifies the ability of drugs to promote changes in gene expression as well as in some, but not necessarily all, drug-induced behavioral effects. These actions of HAT and HDAC pharmacological inhibitors may arise from a complex pattern of genomic and non-genomic effects which cannot be easily dissociated and probably overlap.

Collectively, these data suggest that histone acetylation is involved, at least, in the non-homeostatic neuroplastic mechanisms underlying the development and maintenance of at least some features of addictive behavior. A major challenge for future studies is the attempt to translate this basic knowledge into suitable alternative therapeutic strategies in the treatment and management of the addicted patient.

4.4.2. DNA Methylation

DNA methylation is the most stable epigenetic modification regulating the transcriptional status of mammalian genomes. Accordingly, DNA methylation is an interesting candidate to be involved in at least some enduring forms of neural plasticity. Initial evidence seems to support this idea, although just as in the case of histone modifications, this research has begun only recently, and a general picture of the involvement of DNA methylation in drug abuse and addictive behavior has yet to emerge.

From a mechanistic point of view, methylation occurs when a methyl group is added to position 5 of the cytosine pyrimidine ring in a reaction catalyzed by a group of enzymes called DNA methyltransferases (DNMTs). This mainly takes place when a cytosine is located next to a guanine in the DNA sequence ("CpG" dinucleotides), although cytosine methylation at non-CpG positions has also been reported. The regulatory role of DNA methylation in gene expression is demonstrated by the inverse correlation observed between the level of promoter DNA methylation and the degree of expression of many genes, and it may respond to several environmental signals [83]. These aspects were discussed in Chapter 1.

Drugs of abuse alter the DNA methylation status. Thus, a global enhancement (10%) of DNA methylation levels has been described in alcoholic patients [84]. This global increase likely arises from DNA methylation at gene promoters, which has been documented to occur in response to drug exposure. Thus, for example, methylation increases at the *HERP*, *vasopressin* and *DAT* gene promoters [85-87]. Similarly, increased methylation of some gene promoters has been described in subjects regularly consuming other drugs. Thus, for example, tobacco smokers exhibit hypermethylation of the *p16 tumor suppressor gene* [88] *whereas* methadone-maintained patients show hypermethylation at two binding sites for the transcription factor SP1 at the OPRM1 gene promoter [89]. Taken together, these data indicate that chronic drug exposure enhances global levels of DNA methylation, which may arise from similar changes at specific gene promoters.

However, the effects of chronic drug exposure on DNA methylation are more complex and not fully understood. Again, global measurements might not reveal the functional significance of a particular epigenetic modification. Thus, for example, a reduction (rather than an increase) in methylation has been found at the promoter of the gene MAO-B [90], which indicates that drugs of abuse might promote opposite patterns of DNA methylation to regulate different genes. In other cases, the effects of drug exposure on DNA methylation might be dependent on other factors, such as gender or particular variants of a gene [91]. Finally, it is also important to note that increased or decreased DNA methylation levels do not always translate into the changes at the mRNA or protein that one would expect. For instance, DNA hypermethylation at the HERP gene is accompanied with reduced HERP mRNA levels [85]. However, despite similar hypermethylation of the SNCA (Alpha Synuclein) gene in alcohol-dependent patients [92], SNCA mRNA and protein levels were enhanced, rather than decreased [84, 94]. Further, some limitations of human studies need to be taken into account when considering possible implications. Even for the same individual, epigenetic modifications vary widely from one tissue/cell lineage to another [95]. Additionally, the few sources of DNA that are readily available (*e.g.* lymphocytes) do not usually include the tissue of interest (in this case, neural). On the other hand, many of the factors that could affect DNA samples from drug abuse/addiction patients are difficult to control. Thus, for example, since most of those studies are conducted in patients subjected to therapeutic interventions, it is hard to dissociate the effects of drug exposure from those derived from detoxification or subsequent medical treatments, or indeed from events occurring before drug consumption [89]. Similarly, the correlational nature of this kind of studies does not allow the establishment of causal relationships between different findings, which can only be integrated according to post hoc explanations [96].

Evidence from animal studies might surmount some of those limitations, and thus corroborate the findings of human studies and provide explanations of how drug exposure triggers neuroplastic processes involving DNA methylation. Indeed, experiments in mice have confirmed that hypomethylation at the MAO-B gene promoter in current and long-term abstinent smokers is produced by one or more of the components of tobacco smoke [90]. Similarly, preclinical studies have shown that alcohol exposure reduces methylation levels at introns 1 and 2 of the NR2B gene, leading to an enhancement of the expression of this NMDA-glutamate receptor subunit in cortical neurons [97].

Drug exposure results in significant changes in the expression of DNA methylating enzymes, thus providing a possible mechanism whereby drugs of abuse might modulate DNA methylation. However, some of the results are contradictory and further exploration is required to elucidate the reasons for the apparent discrepancies. Thus, Numachi *et al.* (2007) observed that both acute and repeated methamphetamine administration alters Dnmt1 mRNA levels, and that the direction of these changes depends on the rat strain examined and the brain area considered [98]. Similarly, nicotine decreases the expression of this enzyme [99]. Conversely, other studies have reported that cocaine exposure does not modify Dnmt1 levels, though it might alter the expression of other DNMTs, such as Dnmt3a and Dnmt3b [100, 101]. Again, despite the discrepancies between these studies they both report that during early cocaine withdrawal (1.5 - 3 hours) the mRNA levels of Dnmt3a increased, and were either normalized [100] or downregulated [101] 24 hours after the cessation of cocaine administration. Future research may clarify these discrepancies and elucidate the participation of DNMT3a in addictive behavior (for a recent prospective comment, see [102]).

Reports assessing the functional consequences of DNMT inhibition highlight the role of these enzymes in the behavior observed after repeated drug administration, although they do not examine the mechanisms involved. Thus, LaPlant *et al.* (2010) have shown that repeated systemic administration of methionine (a methyl donor) results in a dramatic decrease of CPP, whereas the intra-accumbal administration of RG108 (a non-nucleoside inhibitor of DNA methylation) results in a moderate enhancement cocaine-induced CPP and locomotor sensitization [101]. In the same study a selective suppression of Dnmt3A (achieved by the administration of an adeno-associated virus vector expressing the recombinase Cre in the NAcc of mice homozygous for a loxP-flanked Dnmt3a gene) but not Dnmt1, reduced DNA methylation levels as well as potentiated cocaine-induced CPP. Conversely, accumbal Dnmt3a overexpression (produced by herpes-simplex virus vector) had the opposite functional consequences. Therefore, taken together, the results of LaPlant *et al.* (2010) suggest that the degree of cocaine-induced CPP is inversely related to methylation levels in the NAcc, also revealing a predominant role of DNMT3A [101]. However, evidence from other studies indicates that the participation of DNA-methylation in the behavioral effects observed after repeated administration of psychostimulants is more complex. Thus, Anier *et al.* (2010) reported that intracerebroventricular administration of the DNMT inhibitor zebularine resulted in decreased, rather than increased, cocaine-induced locomotor sensitization [100]. Similarly, Han *et al.* (2010) have shown that administration of another DNMT inhibitor (5-aza-2-deoxycytidine; 5-AZA) can block cocaine-induced CPP [103]. These discrepancies might be reconciled if DNMT regulation of DNA-methylation were found to have distinct roles in different brain areas, which then had different consequences for the behavioral effects observed after repeated drug administration. Indeed, the study by Han *et al.* showed that selective administration of 5-AZA in the hippocampus and prelimbic cortex prevents the acquisition and expression of cocaine-induced CPP, respectively.

Another aspect of the involvement of DNA methylation processes in drug-induced neuroplasticity has been explored by the study of proteins that preferentially bind to methylated DNA, such as the methyl CpG-binding protein-2 (MeCP2). MeCP2 was initially characterized as part of a larger transcriptional repressor complex (which includes HDACs, HMTs and the co-repressor Sin3a) that binds to methylated CpG sites. Its overexpression, as well as any loss of its function, results in severe neurological alterations, such as the Rett syndrome [104]. However, more recent evidence suggests that it also binds to non-methylated DNA and that, at least in some cases [106], MeCP2 might dampen transcriptional noise genome-wide in a DNA methylation-dependent manner [105] and promote gene transcription. Thus, the molecular actions of MeCP2 in adult neural cells seem highly complex, including a regulatory role in long- and short-term plasticity. But it is becoming increasingly clear that, through these actions, this protein regulates learning/memory processes [107].

Again, the similarity between the neuroplastic changes underlying these phenomena and some aspects of addictive behavior has prompted interest in MeCP2 (and other methyl-binding proteins) in the drug addiction field. Thus, Cassel *et al.* (2006) demonstrated that repeated cocaine exposure leads to enhanced expression of MeCP2 and other methyl-binding proteins in GABAergic neurons of brain areas such as the caudate-putamen, the frontal cortex, and the dentate gyrus [58]. Similarly, Deng *et al.* (2010) observed that amphetamine administration enhances MeCP2 phosphorylation at serine 421 in GABAergic neurons of the NAcc [108]. However, the effects of cocaine on MeCP2 levels are complex and might be modulated by several factors. Im *et al.* (2010), observed an increase in MeCP2 expression in the dorsal, but not the ventral, striatum in rats with extended (but not limited) access to cocaine self-administration [109]. Further, under the same conditions, these authors observed a decrease in MeCP2 expression in the prefrontal cortex, which contrasts with the findings of Cassel *et al.* (2006) [58]. On the other hand, as mentioned above, the functional consequences of such a global enhancement of MeCP2 levels are difficult to predict, even within a restricted cell population. Indeed, another recent study [100] has shown that repeated cocaine administration results in increased MeCP2 binding to the promoters of some genes (such as *PP1*) while its binding to other gene promoters (such as *FosB*) is simultaneously decreased.

Other authors have tried to obtain more direct information about the role of MeCP2 in addictive behavior by directly manipulating its levels in the adult brain. Thus, Im *et al.* (2010) showed that knockdown of MeCP2 in the striatum resulted in a reduction of cocaine self-administration (in rats with extended access to cocaine) [109]. Similarly, *Mecp2* hypomorphic mutant mice (*Mecp2*[3y] mice) display reduced CPP and locomotor sensitization in response to repeated amphetamine injections [109]. However, when the same authors sought to complement their findings by manipulating MeCP2 levels in the NAcc of adult mice *via* lentivirus vectors, completely opposite results were found. Thus, Deng *et al.* (2010) found that locomotion scores after acute amphetamine administration, as well as the development of locomotor sensitization and CPP observed when this treatment was repeated, were enhanced in mice expressing an shRNA against MeCP2 [108]. Complementarily, when a similar strategy was used to enhance MeCP2 expression, a complete blockade of amphetamine-induced CPP was found. At present, there is no an easy way to reconcile these and other findings [100, 110] or the different mechanisms proposed by each author to account for the multiple roles of MeCP2 in different neurobehavioral effects observed after repeated drug exposure. These mechanisms might include a regulatory role of MeCP2 over *Bdnf* expression levels [109, 110] as well as over some other processes controlling structural forms of neuroplasticity such as spine formation [108]. Although all these studies have provided an important contribution by revealing the participation of MeCP2 in several behavioral and neural effects relevant for drug addiction, the particulars of the concourse of this methyl-binding protein (as well as other DNA-methylation related processes) remain largely unknown (for a more extended comment on this topic, see Feng and Nestler, 2010 [111]).

4.5. EPIGENETICS AND TREATMENT OF ADDICTIVE BEHAVIOR

4.5.1. Current Treatments for Drug Abuse and Drug Addiction

The central hypothesis guiding research in the drug abuse/addiction field is that these phenomena need to be understood in terms of the actions of drugs on the brain's motivational and learning/memory systems [22, 26, 112]. Thus, much of this research has embraced positive reinforcement principles as a general framework. Accordingly, for a long time, unraveling the neural mechanisms underlying the reinforcing (sometimes misleadingly referred to as "rewarding") effects of drugs of abuse was considered the best scientific strategy to understand addiction as well as to develop appropriate pharmacological tools for its treatment [113, 114]. This research has resulted in remarkable advances in defining the primary molecular targets of addictive drugs as well as demonstrating that these drugs act as potent behavioral reinforcers [26]. However, it is much more questionable whether pharmacological treatments to block the reinforcing effects of drugs of abuse are the optimal strategy in the clinical management of addictive behavior. Indeed, it is increasingly acknowledged that therapeutic strategies might depart from a conceptual distinction between drug consumption and drug addiction. Accordingly, since the two phenomena are maintained by separate behavioral and neurobiological mechanisms, the clinical management of addiction can no longer be based on attempts to interfere with drug-induced pharmacological effects at the synaptic level. Interestingly, initial evidence suggests that epigenetic mechanisms might provide new avenues in the treatment of addiction, in the light of recent theoretical perspectives. The data are scarce and consequently this section is mainly devoted to describing how the exploration of epigenetic mechanisms might contribute to the development of more effective therapeutic strategies to help drug-addicted patients.

Drug addiction is currently viewed as the endpoint of a series of transitions (Fig. **2**), from initial voluntary drug use to the loss of control over this behavior, which becomes habitual and ultimately compulsive [22, 112]. The behavioral processes and brain structures governing each stage are different and require a differentiated study and clinical management [22, 114]. Thus, initial drug consumption and its maintenance might be largely understood as deriving from the ability of drugs to act as reinforcers. First, drugs may act as positive reinforcers, then establishing and priming drug-seeking/taking behavioral repertoires [22, 26]. Drugs can also reduce specific needs or drives in negatively reinforced contingencies, a possibility which is likely to grow after prolonged drug exposure, when drug taking can partially aim to prevent withdrawal [23]. At this initial behavioral stage, antagonizing the ability of drugs of abuse to act as positive reinforcers or trying to replace them by low potency or medically safer compounds might result in a reduction of drug-seeking/taking behavior. Although it has demonstrated some clinical usefulness, this kind of treatment is only available for some drugs, has a high rejection/desertion rate and often fails to prevent relapse [15, 115].

The failure of current pharmacological treatments in promoting long-term abstinence or preventing relapse is probably due to Pavlovian conditioning-related phenomena that develop concurrently to initial drug self-administration [116, 117]. Thus, in both positive and negatively reinforced situations, environmental stimuli become associated with drugs and thus acquire incentive-motivational properties [22, 118]. These drug-associated stimuli (cues) prompt drug-seeking behavior and evoke memories of the drug, precipitating relapse or inducing craving if the drug cannot be consumed [114]. Drug cues might replace the drug itself in associative learning contingencies, thus becoming 'conditioned

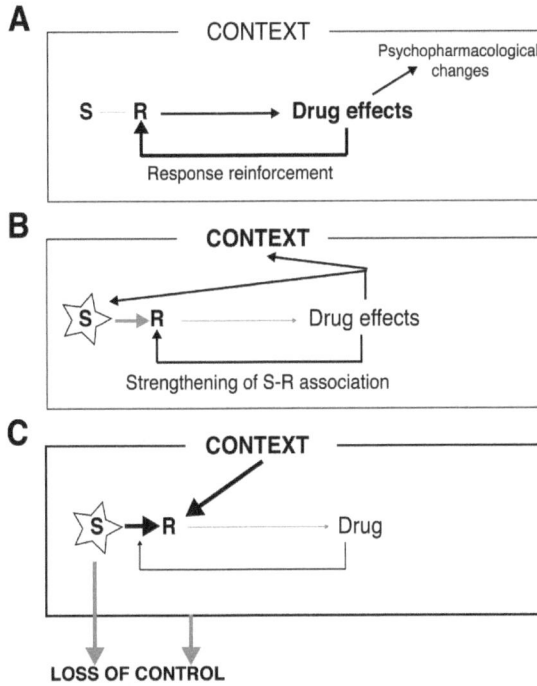

Figure 2: Schematic representation of the mechanisms responsible of the individuals' behavior across the main stages in the transitions towards addiction. Initial drug consumption (A) can be understood as goal-oriented behavior in which the effects of drugs are foreseen and voluntarily pursued. Each drug consumption episode increases the probability of emitting drug-related behavior on future occasions by positive or negative reinforcement processes. Over time, drug consumption might become habitual (B). When drug-related responses become behavioral habits they are largely independent of their consequences (magnitude or quality of the psychopharmacological effects of the drugs) but rather triggered automatically by drug-associated stimuli (drug cues) and associated contexts. Drug cues acquire incentive motivational properties, and thus attract individuals towards them, and each new drug consumption episode increases its incentive force and reinforces its ability to act as occasion-setters (triggering drug-taking behavior) or conditioned reinforcers able to sustain drug-seeking repertoires when drugs are not readily available. Finally, some individuals undergo one further transition and reach the addicted state (C). The most prominent feature of this stage is the individual's loss of control over his or her own behavior, which is precipitated by the sensitization of the incentive motivation acquired by drug cues as well as by reduced prefrontal executive functioning. Those (and probably other mechanisms) translate into reduced willpower and a diminished ability to refrain from drug seeking/taking behavior despite voluntary attempts to do so, especially in the presence of drug cues/drug-associated cues. At this point, behavior is not just automatic (as in behavioral habits) but also compulsive. S=Stimulus; R=Response.

reinforcers' able to sustain drug seeking behavior in the absence of drug availability. Further, as these behaviors are assiduously repeated, the learned association between drug cues and drug-related responses is reinforced. That is, by promoting an increased associative strength of specific stimuli-response contingencies *via* a process that does not necessarily involve learning about the reinforcer itself, drugs (or drug cues) can enhance the storage of information about situations in which they occur, biasing the choice of particular responses, increasing the probability of their emission and facilitating the establishment behavioral habits [112]. In this way, behavior evolves from being a declarative process arising from the coordinated activity of a system involving the ventral striatum and prefrontal regions into a behavioral habit mainly controlled by the dorsal striatum, working memory circuitry and, probably, the cerebellum [15, 22, 119]. As a result, drug seeking and taking behaviors become progressively more independent of their consequences and turn into automatic responses to drug-associated cues acting as 'occasion setters'. Thus, whereas initial drug consumption is motivated by the primary reinforcing effects of these substances, whose psychoactive (*e.g.* "hedonic") effects are foreseen and voluntarily pursued, at the habit stage drug-related behaviors are no longer maintained by their consequences and become largely insensitive to the reinforcers' devaluation or even suppression. Accordingly, when drug consumption has become habitual, pharmacological strategies aimed to block or replace the drugs' psychopharmacological effects might already be largely ineffective.

From habitual drug consumption a relatively small subset of individuals still undergo one more behavioral transition and reach the "addicted state", at which stage drug seeking/taking behavior becomes compulsive. Thus, addictive behavior is not just automatic (as in behavioral habits) but uncontrollable, despite voluntary attempts to restrain it [22, 112, 120-124]. This loss of control may arise from vulnerability traits (*e.g.* impulsivity [125, 126]) as well as from some drug effects that are not exclusively related to their ability to act as reinforcers. In this regard, although there is still debate on their relative contribution to the transition towards addiction, it is generally acknowledged that the inability of addicts to refrain from drug-seeking/taking behavior is attributable to several factors. These include: the progressive sensitization of the incentive value of drug-associated cues [21, 123]; the invigoration of drug-related behavior [27]; the dysregulation of systems involved in the valuation of drugs and natural reinforcers [23]; and neuropathological processes that reduce top-down inhibitory control mechanisms [127, 128].

4.5.2. Novel Treatments for Drug Abuse and Drug Addiction

Regardless of their temporal persistence or functional significance, all the cognitive and behavioral alterations described above derive from the ability of drugs to induce neuroplastic modifications that rely upon changes in gene expression. As mentioned above, emerging evidence suggests that drugs of abuse (like other environmental stimuli) trigger those changes through their ability to, direct or indirectly, recruit complex molecular cascades that include epigenetic mechanisms governing transcriptional processes. Thus, epigenetic marks might store and index complex patterns of gene expression, some of which are finally translated into structural alterations of synaptic connections and macrostructural networks between distant brain areas. Not surprisingly, attending to the behavioral transitions previously explained, addiction has recently been described as "a pathology of staged neuroplasticity" [15]. However, although the description of these forms of drug-induced neuroplasticity might provide a satisfactory (although probably yet incomplete) framework in which to conceive some features of addictive behavior such its temporal persistence, it might be less able to account for its apparent irreversibility. In this regard, recent evidence suggests that drug exposure not only promotes the neuroplastic changes accounting for addictive behaviour, but also reduces the ability of the CNS to revert these changes [24]. Such a reduction might convey the brain into an "anaplastic" state [129, 130], in which drug-induced neuroplastic changes can no longer be reversed, thus locking up the cognitive biases and behavioral repertoires imposed by repeated drug consumption. From this perspective, addiction is a disorder of brain neuroplasticity that is expressed in impairment in the ability to refrain from drug-related behavior, and produces a maladaptive interaction with the environment, including the loss of social compatibility.

Accordingly, the rationale of therapeutic attempts to manage drug-related habits and addictive behavior should focus on the development of therapeutic strategies aimed to prevent, reverse or counteract drug-induced neuroplasticity rather than trying to interfere with the primary reinforcing effects of the drugs of abuse. Attempts to prevent drug-induced neural changes might be clinically unrealistic; as such changes have probably already occurred in individuals seeking treatment. However, developing pharmacological strategies to enhance/restore the plastic capacity lost by neural cells after repeated drug exposure seems more feasible. Such an increase in general neuroplastic capacity might enhance the effectiveness of cognitive/behavioral therapy-based interventions aimed to counteract drug seeking and taking behavior by increasing cognitive flexibility and promoting appropriate decision-making processes. Surprisingly, attempts to identify pharmacological treatments to cope with addiction-related symptoms have largely ignored this possible approach. Indeed, it has been demonstrated that pharmacological and psychological interventions mutually boost their therapeutic value [131, 132]. However, none of the pharmacological agents routinely used in the management of addictive behavior has been specifically developed to maximize the efficacy of the behavioral therapy-based interventions [133].

These psychological therapeutic programs often include interventions aimed to overcome the ability of environmental stimuli to precipitate automatic drug-seeking and taking-related behavior, such as un-reinforced exposure to drug-conditioned stimuli (cues) in an attempt to reduce (*i.e.* extinguish) the addict's conditioned responses to such cues [134-138]. When examined critically (for a meta-analysis, see [139]), cue-exposure treatments are ineffective in the management of addictive behavior, especially in the prevention of relapse episodes. There are multiple reasons for the poor outcome of these interventions, including insufficient knowledge of the optimal conditions to apply extinction-based procedures in the clinical context. However, one reason for the failure of these procedures might be the inherent weakness of extinction as compared to the powerful initial conditioning produced by drugs of abuse. The strength of this initial conditioning relies on the ability of drugs of abuse to act as powerful reinforcers but also, as described above, drugs are potent brain remodelers that trigger several maladaptive processes as well as preventing further neural modifications.

Although preclinical studies on extinction have provided several hints for improving cue-exposure based therapeutic approaches [138, 139], basic research on drug seeking behavior has not devoted enough attention to this topic and it has mainly focused on one of its threats (*i.e.* relapse). Indeed, at the preclinical level, extinction of drug-seeking behavior has largely been considered as "a transition phase" needed to study other phenomena, such as reinstatement, rather than a key aspect of addictive behavior [34]. However, this situation has begun to change, and there is increasing interest in elucidating the molecular substrates of the extinction of maladaptive (*i.e.* drug-seeking) behavior and identifying possible pharmacological agents that could boost the development of extinction after repeated un-reinforced cue exposure.

4.5.2.1. D-Cycloserine

Recent studies have demonstrated that extinction of drug-related behavior can be enhanced pharmacologically [137, 140]. Most of the research has so far focused on the role of glutamatergic receptors and, in particular, the N-methyl-D-aspartate (NMDA) glutamate receptor. Several studies have shown that its partial agonist, D-4-animo-3-isoxazolalidone (D-cycloserine) can facilitate extinction of cocaine- and alcohol-seeking behavior although its ability to reduce reinstatement/relapse-like behavior seems more inconsistent [141-146] Further, other studies have shown that, besides promoting faster and more resistant extinction, D-cycloserine might also reduce the context-dependency that usually presents this phenomenon [147] and that limits its usefulness in the clinical context [139, 148]. These preclinical findings have been followed by clinical trials that have shown that D-cycloserine is useful for augmenting exposure-based therapy (for a recent meta-analysis, see [149]). Therefore, although the use of D-cycloserine for promoting drug abstinence and preventing relapse is problematic, this line of research has demonstrated the enormous potential of using pharmacological strategies that enhance extinction of drug-seeking behavior promoted by unreinforced cue exposure.

4.5.2.2. N-Acetylcysteine

Some of the latest findings regarding a possible therapeutic use of N-acetylcysteine (NAC) in the management of addictive behavior might be interpreted in a similar way. NAC is a cysteine pro-drug that restores basal glutamate levels and prevents increased glutamate during reinstatement by reversing glutamate dysregulation [15, 150-152]. At first, authors assessing the potential usefulness of NAC as an anti-craving compound proposed that these molecular actions could be responsible for the ability of this drug (when administered at the reinstatement test day) to block the re-emergence of previously extinguished drug seeking behavior [151, 153]. However, it has recently been demonstrated that the effects of NAC are much stronger and more durable when it is administered concurrently to un-reinforced cue-exposure [154]. Indeed, when it accompanied extinction sessions, NAC protection outlives NAC bioavailability and promotes a reduction of drug-seeking behavior for weeks after the discontinuation of its administration. This observation, together with the known ability of NAC to improve learning/memory consolidation processes in a wide range of paradigms [155-157], suggests that NAC might enhance the consolidation of extinction-related memories Furthermore, NAC reverses the reduction of brain metaplastic capabilities associated with chronic cocaine administration [24, 158], an effect that might "prepare the ground" for extinction-related re-learning processes . These different mechanisms are not mutually incompatible and they may all contribute to the ability of NAC to reduce drug-seeking behavior. Future research may clarify the mechanisms of NAC cerebral actions but NAC might reduce the probability of relapse, especially if combined with extinction sessions.

4.5.2.3. HDACi

Similarly, in an attempt to promote a more direct intervention in the gene expression changes that support extinction, HDACi have also been used to potentiate the effects of unreinforced cue-exposure. Again, these studies were initiated in the learning/memory field and HDACi were tested as possible pharmacological boosters of the behavioral changes derived from exposure-based psychotherapeutic approaches to treat anxiety-related disorders (reviewed in [159]). However, very recently they have also been tested in the context of drug abuse/addiction research. Thus, the administration of sodium butyrate promotes enhanced extinction of cocaine- [160] as well as morphine- [161] induced CPP. Interestingly, these effects were observed when sodium butyrate was given immediately after each extinction session, but not when it was given10 hours later or in the absence of re-exposure to the conditioning apparatus. These additional observations not only rule out several possible confounding factors (*i.e.* a general disruptive effect on memory) but also, together with short-half life of HDACi such as sodium butyrate, they increase their potential usefulness in the clinical settings. Thus, these pharmacological agents could be administered after successful un-reinforced cue-exposure sessions and "selectively" potentiate the consolidation of this re-learning process.

Furthermore, in these studies [160, 161] HDAC inhibition increased the rate of extinction, as reflected in faster loss of preference for the drug-paired compartment of the CPP apparatus, but also its resistance to external influences. Thus, mice or rats treated with sodium butyrate after each extinction session were resistant to the ability of drug eliminating to reinstate preference for that compartment (a phenomenon that was observed in vehicle-treated subjects). These combined effects on rate and resistance are consistent with the idea that sodium butyrate enhanced extinction of the cocaine-induced place preference, perhaps by making the alternative "no-response" (loss of preference) as powerful as the initial conditioned approach/preference response towards cues established by repeated drug administration. Future studies should explore whether the HDACi-potentiated "no-response" learnt during extinction training is as persistent as those promoted by drugs of abuse. Future research should also attempt to establish whether the extinction responses also remain preeminent over drug habits long after the cessation of the extinction training phase.

While these studies have shown that HDACi (or at least sodium butyrate) might reduce drug-seeking behavior, they did not investigate the possible mechanisms responsible. However, considering that extinction is a new learning event and not an "unlearning" or "forgetting" event, those findings might be viewed in the same perspective as those showing that HDAC inhibition facilitates the acquisition of several responses, including drug-conditioned preference. These authors have almost unanimously suggested that HDACi might increase access to transcription factors, thereby increasing transcription and translation necessary for memory consolidation (for example see [35, 50, 162-164]). Because similar consolidation mechanisms have been shown to operate during extinction, one possibility is that the ability of HDACi to enhance extinction might also depend on its facilitating effects on gene transcription. At present there is no direct support for such a proposal but it seems consistent with the restricted time-window within which HDACi need to be administered in order to potentiate the effects of un-reinforced cue-exposure [160]. Future studies should explore the mechanisms underlying the ability of HDACi to reduce drug-seeking behavior, but they might be used in coadjunctive treatment of exposure-based psychotherapeutical interventions in clinical settings, as observed in drug habits and cognitive biases.

In the same way, other behavioral consequences observed after the administration of HDACi suggest that they might be used in the clinical management of drug abuse/addiction. As already mentioned, one difficulty in the treatment of addictive behavior is the subjects' reduced ability to control their own behavior. This is due not only to the strong appeal of the drug cues, but also to the reduced chances of executive functions to interrupt the behavioral processes triggered by these cues. Consequently, increasing cognitive flexibility and restoring cognitive control over drug-seeking habits has become a major challenge [15]. Several preclinical studies have shown that HDACi might restore several cognitive capabilities, including executive functions and general cognitive flexibility (*e.g.* reversal learning), in subjects bearing several kinds of brain insults or neurological conditions [165-169]. The same treatment also might restore ethanol-related brain damage by reversing ethanol effects in neural stem cell differentiation [170]. Therefore, although it remains to be established experimentally, the administration of HDACi could be a promising approach when trying to increase cognitive flexibility and restore appropriate decision-making processes in drug addicts. Thus, for example (taking into account that the administration of HDACi might reverse several neuroplastic processes associated with DNA and histone methylation), it is tempting to speculate that these pharmacological compounds could reverse the long-lasting attentional deficits and gene-expression changes supported by reduced H3K9 and H3K27 trimethylation levels observed in the prefrontal cortex of rats treated with cocaine during adolescence [171].

Still other effects observed after HDACi administration suggest that these compounds might be interesting tools in the clinical management of drug abusers or addicted patients. Some of these effects might result not from interference with addictive behavior but rather from the improvement of other psychological alterations that complicate treatment (psychiatric co-morbidity). Thus, for example, sodium butyrate reduces some forms of anxiety-like and depression-like behavior [172]. Similarly, withdrawal from chronic alcohol exposure is accompanied by increased HDAC activity, amygdalar *NPY* expression and anxiety–like behaviors, and the HDACi TSA reversed all those effects [56]. At present, it is unclear which neurobiological mechanisms and behavioral processes could be affected by a single HDACi administration shortly before subjects were tested for anxiety-like behavior, but such a reduction of ethanol-withdrawal anxiety might be interesting from a clinical point of view. Attending to the significant co-morbidity of depression and drug abuse/addiction, it should also be highlighted the antidepressant effects of several HDACi [172, 173] as well as the broad use of the HDACi valproic acid as a mood stabilizer in the treatment of several psychiatric diseases [174-176].

In summary, although interest in the possible use of HDACi in the clinical management of drug abuse and addictive behavior is only recent, there are many reasons to suppose that such research will be fruitful. First, the ability of HDACi to enhance the consolidation of learning/memory processes might be a very powerful complement to behavioral interventions such as those based on un-reinforced cue-exposure. This therapeutic strategy seems to be in line with the current views of addiction, which broadly agree that a possible blockade of the drugs' primary psychopharmacological effects is not an adequate strategy to promote protracted abstinence and prevent relapse (the two major difficulties in treatment). Further, this kind of approach seems to combine the "content specificity" that only psychological interventions can achieve with the ability of HDACi to promote long-lasting neuroplastic changes, thus maximizing the benefits of psychotherapeutic- and pharmacological-based treatments. However, HDACi might help behavioral interventions through mechanisms and processes other than enhancing the consolidation of the learning promoted by those activities. Indeed, taking into account the ability of HDACi to increase cognitive abilities after a wide range of brain insults, compounds of this kind might increase the efficacy of psychological interventions by restoring the brain's neuroplastic capabilities reduced by repeated drug use. In this way, HDACi might be promising tools when trying to reverse the anaplastic state that characterizes addiction and triggers compulsive relapse of drug seeking and taking. More specifically, HDACi might promote the cognitive flexibility needed to ensure the success of neuropsychological and behavioral therapy aimed to restore executive functions and proper decision-making processes. Thus, by promoting cognitive flexibility HDACi can potentially increase the penetrability of cognitive and behavioral interventions but also, following a slightly different treatment strategy and HDACi administration regimen, these compounds could boost the consolidation of the benefits achieved during those psychotherapeutic sessions. Finally, when considering the use of HDACi in the treatment of the addicted patient, other effects of at least some HDACi might also be considered. These other effects, such as their possible ameliorating effects of anxiety- and depression-related symptoms, are not directly aimed to reduce addictive behavior but rather to reduce or eliminate some obstacles often found in its treatment. All these HDACi characteristics, together with the fact that several of them are safe and already being tested in human clinical trials (due to their application in the treatment of other diseases such as cancer), should fuel the research aimed to explore whether HDACi (and perhaps other pharmacological compounds able to alter epigenetic mechanisms) might provide new avenues in the clinical management of addictive behavior.

ACKNOWLEDGEMENTS

This study was supported by a grant from Ministerio de Educación y Ciencia (CYCIT) Programa de Investigación Fundamental PSI2008-0131/PSIC awarded to M. Miquel and a grant from Oficina de Investigación Sanitaria (Generalitat Valenciana) AP2377/11 awarded to C. Sanchis-Segura.

REFERENCES

[1]   Newman TK, Syagailo YV, Barr CS, Wendland JR, Champoux M, Graessle M, *et al.* Monoamine-oxidase A gene promoter variation and rearing experience influences aggressive behavior in rhesus monkeys. Biol Psychiatry 2005; 57:167-72.
[2]   Schwandt ML, Lindell SG, Sjöberg RL, Chisholm KL, Higley JD, Suomi SJ, *et al.* Gene-environment interactions and response to social intrusión in male and female rhesus macaques. Biol Psychiatr 2010; 67: 323-30.
[3]   Schwandt ML, Lindell SG, Chen S, Higley JD, Suomi SJ, Heilig M, *et al.* Alcohol response and consumption in adolescente rhesus macaques: life history and genetic influences. Alcohol 2010; 44:67-80
[4]   Sillaber I, Rammes G, Zimmermann S, Mahal B, Zieglgänsberger W, Wurst W, *et al.* Enhanced and delayed stress-induced alcohol drinking in mice lacking functional CRH1 receptors. Science 2002; 296: 931-3.
[5]   Hsieh J, Gage FH. Epigenetic control of neural stem cell fate. Curr Opin Genet Dev 2004; 14: 461-469.
[6]   Borrelli E, Nestler EJ, Allis CD, Sassone-Corsi P. Decoding the epigenetic language of neuronal plasticity Neuron 2008; 60: 961-74

[7]   Fraga MF, Ballestar E, Paz MF, Ropero S, Setien F, Ballestar ML, *et al.* Epigenetic differences arise during lifetime of monozygotic twins. Proc Natl Acad Sci U S A 2005;102: 10604-9.

[8]   Eggeret F, Liang GN, Aparicio A, Jones PA. Epigenetics in human disease and prospects of epigenetic therapy. Nature 2004; 429: 457-63.

[9]   Whitelaw NC, Whitelaw E. How lifetime shapes epigenotypes within and across generations. *Hum. Mol. Genet* 2006; 15: R131-7.

[10]   Jirtle RL, Skinner MK. Environmental epigenomics and diseases susceptibility. Nat Rev Gen 2007; 8: 253-62.

[11]   McClung CA, Nestler EJ. Neuroplasticity mediated by altered gene expression. Neuropsychopharmacology 2008; 33: 3-17.

[12]   Turner BM. Cellular memory and the histone code. Cell 2002; 111: 285-291.

[13]   Barco A, Bailey CH, Kandel ER Common molecular mechanisms in explicit and implicit memory. J Neurochem 2006; 97: 1520–33.

[14]   Nestler EJ, Barrot M, DiLeone RJ, Eisch AJ, Gold SJ, Monteggia LM. Neurobiology of depression. Neuron 2002; 34: 13-25.

[15]   Kalivas PW and O'Brien C. Drug addiction as a pathology of staged neuroplasticity Neuropsychopharmacology 2008; 33: 166-180

[16]   Robinson, T.E. and Kolb, B. Structural plasticity associated with exposure to drugs of abuse. Neuropharmacology 2004; 47: 33–46

[17]   Beitner-Johnson D, Guitart X, Nestler EJ. Neurofilament proteins and the mesolimbic dopamine system common regulation by chronic morphine and chronic cocaine the rat ventral tegemental area. J Neurosci 1992; 12: 2165-76

[18]   Sklair-Tavron L, Shi WX, Lane SB, Harris HW, Bunney BS, Nestler EJ. Chronic morphine induces visible changes in the morphology of mesolimbic dopamine neurons. Proc Natl Acad Sci 1996; 93: 11202–7.

[19]   Stuber GD, Hopf FW, Tye KM, Chen BT, Bonci A. Neuroplastic alterations in the limbic system following cocaine or alcohol exposure Curr Top Behav Neurosci 2010; 3: 3-27.

[20]   Russo SJ, Dietz DM, Dumitriu D, MorrisonJH, Malenka RC, Nestler EJ. The addicted synapse: mechanisms of synaptic and structural plasticity in nucleus accumbens. Trend Neurosci 2010; 33: 267-76

[21]   Robinson TE, Berridge KC. Addiction. Annu Rev Psychol 2003; 54: 25-53

[22]   Everitt EJ and Robbins TW. Systems of reinforcement for drug addiction: from actions to habits to compulsion. Nat Neurosci Rev 2005; 8: 1481-9

[23]   Koob GF. Neurobiological substrates for the dark side of compulsivity in addiction. Neuropharmacology 2009; 56: 18-31.

[24]   Moussawi K, Pacchioni A, Moran AM, Olive MF, Gass JT, Lavin A, *et al.* N-Acetylcysteine reverses cocaine-induced metaplasticity Nat Neurosci 2009; 12: 182-189.

[25]   Lee BR and Dong Y. Cocaine-induced metaplasticity in the nucleus accumbens: Silent synapse and beyond. Neuropharmacology; published online 2011, 21232547.

[26]   Hyman SE, Malenka RC, Nestler EJ. Neural mechanisms of addiction: the role of reward-related learning and memory. Ann Rev Neurosci 2006; 29: 565-98

[27]   Salamone JD, Correa M, Mingote S, Weber SM. Nucleus accumbens dopamine and the regulation of effort in food-seeking behavior: implications for studies of natural motivation, psychiatry, and drug abuse. J Pharmacol Exp Ther 2003; 305: 1-8.

[28]   Li TK, Volkow N. The neuroscience of addiction. Nat Neurosci 2005; 8: 1429–30.

[29]   Jage J. Opioid tolerance and dependence: do they matter? Eur J Pain 2005; 9:157-62.

[30]   O'Brien CP. Benzodiazepine use, abuse, and dependence. J Clin Psychiatry 2005; 66: 28–33.

[31]   McLellan AT, Lewis DC, O'Brien CP, Kleber HD. Drug dependence, a chronic medical illness: implications for treatment, insurance, and outcomes evaluation. JAMA 2000; 284:1689–95.

[32]   Chao J, Nestler EJ. Molecular neurobiology of drug addiction. Annu Rev Med 2004; 55:113–32

[33]   Olmstead MC. Animal models of drug addiction: Where do we go from here?. Q J Exp Psychol 2006; 59: 625-53.

[34]   Sanchis-Segura C, Spanagel R. Behavioural assessment of drug reinforcement and addictive features in rodents: an overview. Addict Biol 2006; 11: 2-38.

[35]   Kumar A, Choi KH, Renthal W, Tsankova NM, Theobald DE, Truong HT, *et al.* Chromatin remodeling is a key mechanism underlying cocaine-induced plasticity in striatum. Neuron 2005; 48:3 03–14.

[36]   Levine AA; Guan Z, Barco A, Xu S, Kandel ER, Schwartz JH. CREB-binding protein controls response to cocaine by acetylating histones at the fosB promoter in the mouse striatum. Proced Nat Acad Sci 2005; 102:19186-91.

[37]   Renthal W and Nestler EJ. Epigenetic mechanisms in drug addiction. Trends Mol Med 2008; 14: 341-50

[38]   Renthal W, Kumar A, Xiao G, Wilkinson M, Covington HE 3rd, Maze I, *et al.* Genome-wide analysis of chromatin regulation by cocaine reveals a role for sirtuins. Neuron 2009; 62: 335-48.

[39]   Esteve PO, Chin HG, Smallwood A, Feehery GR, Gangisetty O, Karpf AR , *et al.* Direct interaction between DNMT1 and G9a coordinates DNA and histone methylation during replication. Genes Dev 2006; 20: 3089-103.

[40]   Epsztejn-Litman S, Feldman N, Abu-Remaileh M, Shufaro Y, Gerson A, Ueda J, *et al. De novo* DNA methylation promoted by G9a prevents reprogramming of embryonically silenced genes. Nat Str Mol Biol 2008; 15: 1176-83.

[41]   McClung CA, Nestler EJ. Regulation of gene expression and cocaine reward by CREB and DeltaFosB. Nat Neurosci 2003; 6:1208-15.

[42]   Maze I, Covington HE 3rd, Dietz DM, LaPlant Q, Renthal W, Russo SJ, *et al.* Essential role of the histone methyltransferase G9a in cocaine-induced plasticity. Science 2010; 327: 213-6.

[43]   McClung CA, Ulery PG, Perrotti LI, Zachariou V, Berton O, Nestler EJ. DeltaFosB: a molecular switch for long-term adaptation in the brain. Brain Res Mol Brain Res 2004; 132:146-50.

[44]   Nestler EJ. Transcriptional mechanisms of addiction: role of DeltaFosB. Philos Trans R Soc Lond B Biol Sci 2008; 363: 3245-55

[45]   Kelz MB, Chen J, Carlezon WA Jr, Whisler K, Gilden L, Beckmann AM, *et al.* Expression of the transcription factor deltaFosB in the brain controls sensitivity to cocaine. Nature 1999; 401: 272-6.

[46]   Brami-Cherrier K, Lavaur J, Pagès C, Arthur JS, Caboche J Glutamate induces histone H3 phosphorylation but not acetylation in striatal neurons: role of mitogen- and stress-activated kinase-1. J Neurochem 2007; 101: 697-708.

[47]   Kouzarides T. Chromatin modifications and their function. Cell 2007; 128: 693-705

[48] Brami-Cherrier K, Roze E, Girault JA, Betuing S, Caboche J. Role of the ERK/MSK1 signalling pathway in chromatin remodelling and brain responses to drugs of abuse. J Neurochem 2009; 108: 1323-35.

[49] Brami-Cherrier K, Valjent E, Hervé D, Darragh J, Corvol JC, Pages C, *et al.* Parsing molecular and behavioral effects of cocaine in mitogen- and stress-activated protein kinase-1-deficient mice. J Neurosci 2005; 25:11444-54.

[50] Sanchis-Segura C, Lopez-Atalaya JP, Barco A. Selective boosting of transcriptional and behavioral responses to drugs of abuse by histone deacetylase inhibition. Neuropsychopharmacology 2009; 3: 2642-54.

[51] Stipanovich A, Valjent E, Matamales M, Nishi A, Ahn JH, Maroteaux M, *et al.* A phosphatase cascade by which rewarding stimuli control nucleosomal response. Nature 2008; 453: 879-84.

[52] Lee YJ, Shukla SD. Histone H3 phosphorylation at serine 10 and serine 28 is mediated by p38 MAPK in rat hepatocytes exposed to ethanol and acetaldehyde. Eur J Pharmacol 2007; 573: 29-38

[53] Cheung P, Tanner KG, Cheung WL, Sassone-Corsi P, Denu JM, Allis CD. Synergistic coupling of histone H3 phosphorylation and acetylation in response to epidermal growth factor stimulation. Mol Cell 2000; 5:905-15.

[54] Bertran-Gonzalez J, Håkansson K, Borgkvist A, Irinopoulou T, Brami-Cherrier K, Usiello A, *et al.* Histone H3 phosphorylation is under the opposite tonic control of dopamine D2 and adenosine A2A receptors in striatopallidal neurons. Neuropsychopharmacology 2009; 34:1710-20

[55] Kim JS, Shukla SD. Acute *in vivo* effect of ethanol (binge drinking) on histone H3 modifications in rat tissues. Alcohol Alcohol 2006; 41: 126-30

[56] Pandey SC, Ugale E, Zhang H, Tang L, Prakash A. Brain chromatin remodeling: a novel mechanism of alcoholism. J Neuroci 2008; 28: 3729-37.

[57] Shen HY, Kalda A, Yu L, Ferrara J, Zhu J, Chen JF. Additive effects of histone deacetylase inhibitors and amphetamine on histone H4 acetylation, cAMP responsive element binding protein phosphorylation and DeltaFosB expression in the striatum and locomotor sensitization in mice. Neuroscience 2008; 157: 644-55.

[58] Cassel S, Carouge D, Gensburger C, Anglard P, Burgun C, Dietrich JB, *et al.* Fluoxetine and cocaine induce the epigenetic factors MeCP2 and MBD1 in adult rat brain. Mol Pharm 2006; 70: 487-92

[59] Pascual M, Boix J, Felipo V, Guerri C. Repeated alcohol administration during adolescence causes changes in the mesolimbic dopaminergic and glutamatergic systems and promotes alcohol intake in the adult rat. J Neurochem 2009; 108: 920-31.

[60] Renthal W and Nestler EJ. Histone acetylation in drug addiction. Semin Cell Dev Biol 2009; 20: 387-94.

[61] Renthal W, Carle TL, Maze I, Covington HE 3rd, Truong HT, Alibhai I, *et al.* Delta FosB mediates epigenetic desensitization of the c-fos gene after chronic amphetamine exposure. J Neurosci 2008; 28: 7344-9.

[62] Freeman WM, Patel KM, Brucklacher RM, Lull ME, Erwin M, Morgan D, *et al.* Persistent alterations in mesolimbic gene expression with abstinence from cocaine self-administration. Neuropsychopharmacology 2008; 33: 1807-17.

[63] Park PH, Lim RW, Shukla SD. Involvement of histone acetyltransferase (HAT) in ethanol-induced acetylation of histone H3 in hepatocytes: potential mechanism for gene expression. Am J Physiol Gastrointest Liver Physiol 2005; 289: G1124-36.

[64]   Host L, Dietrich JB, Carouge D, Aunis D, Zwiller J. Cocaine self-administration alters the expression of chromatin-remodelling proteins; modulation by histone deacetylase inhibition. J Psychopharmacol 2011; 25: 222-9.

[65]   Mattson BJ, Bossert JM, Simmons DE, Nozaki N, Nagarkar D, Kreuter JD, *et al.* Cocaine-induced CREB phosphorylation in nucleus accumbens of cocaine-sensitized rats is enabled by enhanced activation of extracellular signal-related kinase, but not protein kinase A. J Neurochem 2005; 95:1481-94.

[66]   Renthal W, Maze I, Krishnan V, Covington HE 3rd, Xiao G, Kumar A, *et al.* Histone deacetylase 5 epigenetically controls behavioral adaptations to chronic emotional stimuli. Neuron 2007; 56: 517-29.

[67]   Sun J, Wang L, Jiang B, Hui B, Lv Z, Ma L. The effects of sodium butyrate, an inhibitor of histone deacetylase, on the cocaine- and sucrose-maintained self-administration in rats. Neurosci Lett 2008; 441: 72-6.

[68]   Wang L, Lv Z, Hu Z, Sheng J, Hui B, Sun J, Ma L. Chronic cocaine-induced H3 acetylation and transcriptional activation of CaMKIIalpha in the nucleus accumbens is critical for motivation for drug reinforcement. Neuropsychopharmacology 2010; 35: 913-28.

[69]   Romieu P, Host L, Gobaille S, Sandner G, Aunis D, Zwiller J. Histone deacetylase inhibitors decrease cocaine but not sucrose self-administration in rats. J Neurosci 2008; 28: 9342-8

[70]   Schroeder FA, Lin CL, Crusio WE, Akbarian S. Antidepressant-like effects of the histone deacetylase inhibitor, sodium butyrate, in the mouse. Biol Psychiatry 2007; 62: 55-64.

[71]   Hui B, Wang W, Li J. Biphasic modulation of cocaine-induced conditioned place preference through inhibition of histone acetyltransferase and histone deacetylase. Saudi Med J 2010; 31: 389-93.

[72]   Pastor V, Host L, Zwiller J, Bernabeu R. Histone deacetylase inhibition decreases preference without affecting aversion for nicotine. J Neurochem 2011; 116: 636-45.

[73]   Bilbao A, Parkitna JR, Engblom D, Perreau-Lenz S, Sanchis-Segura C, Schneider M, *et al.* Loss of the Ca2+/calmodulin-dependent protein kinase type IV in dopaminoceptive neurons enhances behavioral effects of cocaine. Proc Natl Acad Sci U S A 2008; 105: 17549-54.

[74]   Kalda A, Heidmets LT, Shen HY, Zharkovsky A, Chen JF. Histone deacetylase inhibitors modulates the induction and expression of amphetamine-induced behavioral sensitization partially through an associated learning of the environment in mice Behav Brain Res 2007; 181: 76-84.

[75]   Colvis CM, Pollock JD, Goodman RH, Impey S, Dunn J, Mandel G, *et al.* Epigenetic mechanisms and gene networks in the nervous system. J Neurosci 2005; 25: 10379-89.

[76]   Piechota M, Korostynski M, Solecki W, Gieryk A, Slezak M, Bilecki W, *et al.* The dissection of transcriptional modules regulated by various drugs of abuse in the mouse striatum. Genome Biol 2010; 11: R48.

[77]   Zachariou V, Bolanos CA, Selley DE, Theobald D, Cassidy MP, Kelz MB, *et al.* An essential role for DeltaFosB in the nucleus accumbens in morphine action. Nat Neurosci 2006; 9: 205-11

[78]   Andretic R, Chaney S, Hirsh J. Requirement of circadian genes for cocaine sensitization in Drosophila. Science 1999; 285: 1066-8.

[79]   Abarca C, Albrecht U, Spanagel R. Cocaine sensitization and reward are under the influence of circadian genes and rhythm. Proc Natl Acad Sci U S A 2002; 99: 9026-30.

[80]   Wang Y, Krishnan HR, Ghezzi A, Yin JC, Atkinson NS. Drug-induced epigenetic changes produce drug tolerance. Plos Biol 2007; 5: e265

[81]   Glozak MA, Sengupta N. Zhang X, Seto E. Acetylation and deacetylation of non-histone proteins. Gene 2005; 363:15-23.

[82]   Spange S, Wagner T, Heinzel T, Kramer OH. Acetylation of non-histone proteins modulates cellular signalling at multiple levels. Int J Cell Biochem Biol 2009; 41: 185-98.

[83]   Jaenisch R, Bird A. Epigenetic regulation of gene expression: how the genome integrates intrinsic and environmental signals. Nat Genet 2003; 33: 245-54

[84]   Bönsch D, Lenz B, Reulbach U, Kornhuber J, Bleich S. Homocysteine associated genomic DNA hypermethylation in patients with chronic alcoholism. J Neural Transm 2004; 111:1611-6.

[85]   Bleich S, Lenz B, Ziegenbein M, Beutler S, Frieling H, Kornhuber J, *et al.* Epigenetic DNA hypermethylation of the HERP gene promoter induces down-regulation of its mRNA expression in patients with alcohol dependence. Alcohol Clin Exp Res 2006; 30: 587-91

[86]   Hillemacher T, Frieling H, Hartl T, Wilhelm J, Kornhuber J, Bleich S. Promoter specific methylation of the dopamine transporter gene is altered in alcohol dependence and associated with craving. J Psychiatr Res 2009a; 43: 388-92.

[87]   Hillemacher T, Frieling H, Luber K, Yazici A, Muschler MA, Lenz B, *et al.* Epigenetic regulation and gene expression of vasopressin and atrial natriuretic peptide in alcohol withdrawal. Psychoneuroendocrinology 2009; 34: 555-60.

[88]   vonZeidler SV, Miracca EC, Nagai MA, Birman EG. Hypermethtylation of the p16 gene in normal oral mucosa of smokers. Int J Mol Med 2004; 14: 807-11

[89]   Nielsen, DA, Yuzerof V, Hamon S, Jackson C, Ho A, Ott J, *et al.* Increased *OPRM1* DNA methylation in lymphocytes of methadone-maintained former heroin addicts. Neuropsychopharmacology 2009; 34: 867-73.

[90]   Launay JM, Del Pino M, Chironi G, Callebert J, Peoc'h K, Mégnien JL, *et al.* Smoking induces long-lasting effects through a monoamine-oxidase epigenetic regulation. PloS one 2009; 4: 182-95.

[91]   Philibert RA, Gunter TD, Beach SR, Brody GH, Madan A. MAOA methylation is associated with nicotine and alcohol dependence in women. Am J Med Genet B Neuropsychiatr Genet 2008; 147: 565-70.

[92]   Bönsch D, Lenz B, Kornhuber J, Bleisch S. DNA hypermethylation of the alpha synuclein promoter in patients with alcoholism. Neuroport 2005; 16: 167-70

[93]   Bönsch D, Lenz B, Kornhuber J, Bleich S Alpha-synuclein protein levels are increased in alcoholic patients and are linked to craving. *Alcohol Clin Exp Res 2005; 29:763-5*

[94]   Ollikainen M, Smith KR, Joo EJ, Ng HK, Andronikos R, Novakovic B, *et al.* DNA methylation analysis of multiple tissues from newborn twins reveals both genetic and intrauterine components to variation in the human neonatal epigenome. Hum Mol Genet 2010; 19:4176-88.

[95]   Bönsch D, Lenz B, Fiszer R, Frieling H, Kornhuber J, Bleich S. Lowered DNA methyltransferase (DNMT-3b) mRNA expression is associated with genomic DNA hypermethylation in patients with chronic alcoholism. J Neural Transm 2006; 113:1299-304.

[96]   Marutha Ravindran CR, Ticku MK. Changes in methylation pattern of NMDA receptor NR2B gene in cortical neurons after chronic ethanol treatment in mice. Mol Brain Res 2004; 121:19-27.

[97]   Numachi Y, Shen H, Yoshida S, Fujiyama K, Toda S, Matsuoka H, *et al.* Methamphetamine alters expression of DNA methyltransferase 1 mRNA in rat brain. Neurosci Lett 2007; 414: 213-7.

[98]   Satta R, Maloku E, Zhubi A, Pibiri F, Hajos M, Costa E, *et al.* Nicotine decreases DNA methyltransferase 1 expression and glutamic acid decarboxylase 67 promoter methylation in GABAergic interneurons. Proc Natl Acad Sci 2008;   105: 16356-61

[99]   Anier K, Malinovskaja, K, Aonurm-Helm A, Zharkovsky A, Kalda A. DNA methylation regulates cocaine-induced behavioral sensitization in mice. Neuropsychopharmacology 2010; 35: 2540-61.

[100]   LaPlant Q, Vialou V, Covington III HE, Dumitriu D, Feng J, Warren BL, *et al.* Dnmt3a regulates emotional behavior and spine plasticity in the nucleus accumbens. Nat Neurosci 2010; 13: 1137-45.

[101]   Hopf FW, Bonci A. Dnmt3a: Addiction's molecular forget-me-not? Nat Neurosci 2010; 13: 1041- 42.

[102]   Han J, Li Y, Wang D, Wei C, Yang X, Sui N. Effect of 5-aza-2-deoxycytidine microinjecting into hippocampus and prelimbic cortex on acquisition and retrieval of cocaine-induced place preference in C57BL/6 mice. Eur J Pharmacol 2010; 642: 93-8.

[103]   Amir RE, Van den Veyver IB, Wan M, Tran CQ, Francke U, Zoghbi HY. Rett syndrome is caused by mutations in X-linked MeCP2 endoding methyl-CpG-binding protein 2. Nat Genet 1999; 23:185-8.

[104]   Skene PJ, Illingworth RS, Webb S, Kerr AR, James KD, Turner, DJ, *et al.* Neuronal MeCP2 is expressed at near histone-octamer levels and globally alters at the chromatin state. Mol Cell 2009; 41: 185-98.

[105]   Chahrour M, Jung SY, Shaw C, Zhou X, Wong ST, Qin J, *et al.* MeCP2, a key contributor to neurological disease, activates and represses transcription. Science 2008; 320: 1224-9.

[106]   Na ES, Monteggia LM. The role of MeCP2 in CNS development and function. Horm Behav 2011; 59: 364-8.

[107]   Deng JV, Rodriguez RM, Hutchinson AN, Kim I-H, Wetsel WC, West AE. MeCP2 in the nucleus accumbens contributes to neural and behavioral responses to psychostimulants. Nat Neurosci 2010; 13: 1128-1136.

[108]   Im H-I, Hollander JA, Bali P, Kenny PJ. MeCP2 controls BDNF expression and cocaine intake through homeostatic interactions with microRNA-212. Nat Neurosci 2010; 13: 1120-1127.

[109]   Sadri-Vakili G, Kumaresan V, Schmidt HD, Famous KR, Chawla P, Vassoler FM, *et al.* Cocaine-induced chromatin remodeling increased brain-derived neurotrophic factor transcription in the rat medial prefrontal cortex, which alter the reinforcing efficacy of cocaine. J Neurosci 2010; 30:11735-44.

[110]   Feng J, Nestler EJ. MeCP2 and drug addiction. Nat Neurosci 2010; 13: 1039-1041.

[111]   Everitt BJ, Belin D, Economidou D, Pelloux Y, Dalley JW, Robbins TW. Neural mechanisms underlying the vulnerability to develop compulsive drug-seeking habits and addiction. Philos Trans R Soc Lond B Biol Sci 2008; 363: 3125-35

[112]   Wise RA. The neurobiology of craving: Implications for understanding and treatment of addiction. J Abnorm Psychol 1988; 97: 118-132.

[113]   Tiffany ST. A cognitive model of drug urges and drug-use behavior: role of automatic and nonautomatic processes. Psychol Rev 1990; 97: 147-68.

[114]   Dackis CA and O'Brien CP. Cocaine dependence: A disease of the brain's reward centres. J Subst. Abuse treat 2001; 21: 111-17

[115] O' Brien CP, Childress AR, McLellan AT, Ehrman R. Classical conditioning in drug-dependent humans. Ann NY Acad Sci 1992; 654: 400-15.

[116] O'Brien CP, Childress AR, Ehrman R, Robbins SJ. Conditioning factors in drug abuse: Can they explain compulsion? J Psychopharm 1998; 12: 15-22.

[117] White NM, Milner PM. The Psychobiology of reinforcers. Annu Rev Psychol. 1992; 43: 443-71

[118] Miquel M, Toledo R, García LI, Coria-Avila GA, Manzo J. Why should we keep the cerebellum in mind when thinking about addiction? Curr Drug Abuse Rev 2009; 2: 26-40

[119] Koob GF, Le Moal M. Neurobiological mechanisms for opponent motivational processes in addiction. Philos Trans R Soc Lond B Biol Sci 2008; 363: 3113-23.

[120] Koob GF, Le Moal M. Addiction and the brain antireward system. Annu Rev Psychol. 2008; 59: 29-53.

[121] Koob GF, Le Moal M. Drug addiction, dysregulation of reward, and allostasis. Neuropsychopharmacology 2001; 24:97-129.

[122] Robinson TE, Berridge KC. The incentive sensitization theory of addiction: Some current issues. Philos Trans R Soc Lond B Biol Sci 2008; 363: 3137-46.

[123] Bechara A. Decision making, impulse control and loss of willpower to resist drugs: a neurocognitive perspective. Nat Neurosci 2005; 8: 1458-63

[124] Kreek MJ, Nielsen DA, Butelman ER, LaForge KS. Genetic influences on impulsivity, risk taking, stress responsivity and vulnerability to drug abuse and addiction. Nat Neurosci 2005; 8: 1450-7.

[125] Verdejo-Garcia A and Bechara A. A somatic marker theory of addiction. Neuropharmacology 2009; 56: 48-62.

[126] Volkow ND, Fowler JS, Wang GJ. The addicted human brain viewed in the light of imaging studies: brain circuits and treatment strategies. Neuropharmacology 2004; 47: 3-13.

[127] Goldstein RZ, Craig AD, Bechara A, Garavan H, Childress AR, Paulus MP, *et al.* The neurocircuitry of impaired insight in drug addiction. Trends Cogn Sci 2009; 13: 372-80.

[128] Abraham WC. Metaplasticity: tuning synapses and networks for plasticity. Nat Rev Neurosci 2008; 9: 387-391.

[129] Kasanetz F, Deroche-Gamonet V, Berson N, Balado E, Lafourcade M, Manzoni O, *et al.* Transition to addiction is associated with a persistent impairment in synaptic plasticity. Science 2010; 328:1709-12.

[130] Davis M, Barad, M, Otto M, Southwick S. Combining pharmacotherapy with cognitive behavioral therapy: traditional and new approaches J Traum Stress 2006; 19: 571-581

[131] Swift R. Emerging approaches to managing alcohol dependence. Am J Health Syst Pharm 2007; 64: 12-22

[132] Edens E, Massa A, Petrakis I. Novel pharmacological approaches to drug abuse treatment. Curr Top Behav Neurosci 2010; 3: 343-86.

[133] Raw M, Russell MA. Rapid smoking, cue exposure and support in the modification of smoking. Behav Res Ther 1980; 18: 363-72.

[134] Heather N and Bradley BP. Cue exposure as a practical treatment for addictive disorders: Why are we waiting?. Addict Biol 1990; 15: 335-7.

[135] Otto MW, Safren SA and Pollack MH. Internal cue exposure and the treatment of substance use disorders: lessons from the treatment of panic disorder. J Anxiety Disord 2004; 18: 69-87.

[136] Taylor JR, Olausson P, Quinn JJ, Torregrosa MM. Targeting extinction and re-consolidation mechanisms to combat the impact of drug cues on addiction. Neuropharmacology 2009; 56: 186-95.

[137] Conklin CA, Tiffany ST. Cue-exposure treatment: time for change. Addiction 2002; 97:1219-2

[138] Conklin CA, Tiffany ST. Applying extinction research and theory to cue-exposure addiction treatments. Addiction 2002; 97: 155-67.

[139] Kaplan GB, Moore KA. The use of cognitive enhancers in animal models of fear extinction. Pharmacol Biochem Behav 2011; 99: 217-28.

[140] Botreau F, Paolone G, Stewart J. d-Cycloserine facilitates extinction of a cocaine-induced conditioned place preference. Behav Brain Res 2006; 172: 173-8.

[141] Paolone G, Botreau F, Stewart J. The facilitative effects of D-cycloserine on extinction of a cocaine-induced conditioned place preference can be long lasting and resistant to reinstatement. Psychopharmacology 2009; 202: 403-9.

[142] Groblewski PA, Lattal KM, Cunningham CL. Effects of D-cycloserine on extinction and reconditioning of ethanol-seeking behavior in mice. Alcohol Clin Exp Res 2009; 33: 772-82.

[143] Kelley JB, Anderson KL, Itzhak Y. Long-term memory of cocaine-associated context: disruption and reinstatement. Neuroreport 2007; 18: 777-80.

[144] Vengeliene C, Kiefer F, Spanagel R. D-cycloserine facilitates extinction of conditioned alcohol-seeking behaviour in rats. Alcohol Alcohol 2008; 43: 626-9.

[145] Thanos PK, Bermeo C, Wang GJ, Volkow ND. D-cycloserine accelerates the extinction of cocaine-induced conditioned place preference in C57bL/c mice. Behav Brain Res 2009; 199: 345-9.

[146] Torregrosa MM, Sanchez H, Taylor JR. D-cycloserine reduces the context specificity of pavlovian extinction of cocaine cues through actions in the nucleus accumbens. J Neurosci 2010; 30: 526-33.

[147] Bouton ME. Context and behavioral processes in extinction. Learn Mem 2004; 11: 485–494.

[148] Norberg MM, Krystal JH, Tolin DF. A meta-analysis of D-cycloserine and the facilitation of fear extinction and exposure therapy. Biol Psychiatry 2008; 63: 1118–1126

[149] Baker DA, Xi Z, Shen H, Swanson CJ, Kalivas PW. The origin and neuronal function of *in vivo* nonsynaptic glutamate. J Neurosci 2002; 22: 9134-41.

[150] Baker DA, McFarland K, Lake RW, Shen H, Toda S, Kalivas PW. N-acetyl cysteine-induced blockade of cocaine-induced reinstatement. Ann N Y Acad Sci 2003; 1003:349-51.

[151] Kalivas PW The glutamate homeostasis hypothesis of addiction. Nat Rev Neurosci 2009; 10: 561-72.

[152] Kau KS, Madayag A, Mantsch JR, Grier MD, Abdulhameed O, Baker DA. Blunted cystine-glutamate antiporter function in the nucleus accumbens promotes cocaine-induced drug seeking. Neuroscience 2008; 155: 530-37.

[153] Reichel CM, Moussawi K, Phong HD, Kalivas PW, See RE. Chronic N-acetylcysteine during abstinence or extinction following cocaine self-administration produces enduring reductions in drug-seeking. J Pharmacol Exp Ther 2011; 337: 487-93.

[154] Farr SA, Poon HF, Dogrukol-Ak D, Drake J, Banks WA, Eyerman E, *et al.* The antioxidants alpha-lipoic acid and N-acetylcysteine reversememory impairment and brain oxidative stress in aged SAMP8 mice. J Neurochem 2003: 84:1173-83.

[155] Achat-Mendes C, Anderson KL, Itzhak Y. Impairment in consolidation of learned place preference following dopaminergic neurotoxicity in mice is ameliorated by n-acetylcysteine

but not D1 and D2 dopamine receptor agonists. Neuropsychopharmacology 2007; 32: 531-41.

[156] Prakash A, Kumar A. Effect of N-acetyl cysteine against aluminium-induced cognitive dysfunction and oxidative damage in rats. Basic Clin Pharmacol Toxicol 2009; 105: 98-104.

[157] Moussawi K, Zhou W, Shen H, Reichel CM, See RE, Carr DB, *et al.* Reversing cocaine-induced synaptic potentiation provides enduring protection from relapse. Proc Natl Acad Sci USA 2011; 108: 385-90.

[158] Malvaez M, Barrett RM, Wood MA, Sanchis-Segura C. Epigenetic mechanisms underlying extinction of memory and drug-seeking behavior. Mamm Genome 2009; 20: 612-23.

[159] Malvaez M, Sanchis-Segura C, Vo D, Lattal KM, Wood MA. Modulation of chromatin modification facilitates extinction of cocaine-induced conditioned place preference. Biol Psychiatry 2010; 67: 36-43.

[160] Wang, R Zhang Y, Qing H, Liu M, Yang, P. The extinction of morphine-induced conditioned place preference by histone deacetylase inhibition. Neurosci Lett 11; 483: 137-42

[161] Lattal KM, Barrett RM, Wood MA. Systemic or intrahippocampal delivery of histone deacetylase inhibitors facilitates fear extinction. Behav Neurosci 2007; 121: 1125-31.

[162] Bredy TW, Barad M. The histone deacetylase inhibitor valproic acid enhances acquisition, extinction, and reconsolidation of conditioned fear. Learn Mem 2008; 15: 39-45.

[163] Morris MJ, Karra AS, Monteggia LM. Histone deacetylases govern cellular mechanisms underlying behavioral and synaptic plasticity in the developing and adult brain. Behav Pharmacol 2010; 21: 409-19.

[164] Alarcon JM, Malleret G, Touzani K, Vronkaya S, Ishii S, Kandel ER, *et al.* Chromatin acetylation, memory and LTP are impaired in CBP+/- mice: a model for the cognitive deficit in Rubinstein-Taybi syndrome and its amelioraiton. Neuron 2004; 42: 947-59.

[165] Fontán-Lozano A, Romero-Granados R, Troncoso J, Múnera A, Delgado-García JM, Carrión AM. Histone deaceytlase inhibitors improve learning consolidation in young and in KA-induced neurodegeneration and SAMP-8-mutant mice. Mol Cell Neurosci 2008; 39: 193-201.

[166] Dash PK, Orsi SA, Moore AN. Histone deacetylase inhibition combined with behavioral therapy enhances learning and memory following traumatic brain injury. Neuroscience 2009; 163: 1-8.

[167] Kilgore M, Miller CA, Fass DM, Hennig KM, Haggarty SJ, Sweatt JD, *et al.* Inhibitors of class 1 histone deacetylases reverse contextual memory deficits in a mouse model of Alzheimer's disease. Neuropsychopharmacology 2010; 35: 870-80

[168] Ricobaraza A, Cuadrado-Tejedor M, Marco S, Pérez-Otavo I, García-Osta A. Phenylbutyrate rescues dendritic spine loss associated with memory deficits in a mouse model of Alzheimer disease. Hippocampus, published online 2010, 21069780.

[169] Ishii T, Hashimoto E, Ukai W, Tateno M, Yoshinaga T, Ono T, *et al.* Epigenetic regulation in alcohol-related brain damage. Nihon Arukoru Yakubutsu Igakkai Zasshi 2008; 43:705–13

[170] Black YD, Maclaren FR, Naydenov AV, Carlezon WA Jr, Baxter MG, Konradi C. Altered attention and prefrontal cortex gene expression in rats after binge-like exposure to cocaine during adolescence. J Neurosci 2006; 26: 9656-65.

[171] Gundersen BB and Bredy JA. Effects of the histone deacetylase inhibitor sodium butyrate in models of depression and anxiety. Neuropharmacology 2009; 57: 67-74.

[172] Schroeder M, Krebs MO, Bleich S, Frieling H. Epigenetics and depression: current challenges and new therapeutic options. Curr Opin Psychiatry 2010; 23: 588-92.

[173] Tsankova NM, Berton O, Renthal W, Kumar A, Neve RL, Nestler EJ. Sustained hippocampal chromatin regulation in a mouse model of depression and antidepressant action. Nat Neurosci 2006; 9: 519-25.

[174] Adamou M, Puchalska S, Plummer W, Hale AS. Valproate in the treatment of PTSD: systematic review and meta análisis . Curr Med Res Opin 2007; 23: 1285-91.

[175] Amann B, Grunze H, Vieta E, Trimble M. Antiepileptic drugs and mood stability. Clin EEG Neurosci 2007; 38: 116-23

[176] Calabrese JR, Shelton MD, Rapport DJ, Kujawa M, Kimmel SE, Caban S. Current research on rapid cycling bipolar disorder and its treatment. J Affect Disord 2001; 67: 241-55.

CHAPTER 5

Epigenetics of Nutrition

Karen A. Lillycrop[1,*] and Graham C. Burdge[2]

¹School of Biological Sciences, Faculty of Natural and Environmental Sciences, and ²Human Development and Health, Faculty of Medicine, University of Southampton, Southampton, UK

Abstract: Epigenetic processes play a central role in regulating the tissue-specific expression of genes. Alterations in these processes can therefore lead to profound changes in phenotype and have been implicated in the pathogenesis of many human diseases. However, there is now evidence that the epigenome is susceptible to a range of environmental cues such as variations in diet, maternal behaviour or stress during specific developmental periods. The environmental sensitivity of the epigenome has been suggested to reflect an adaptive mechanism, by which the organism can adjust its metabolism and homeostatic systems to suit the environment, in order to aid survival or reproductive success in later life. Inappropriate adaptation has been linked to the development of a range of chronic diseases in later life and has been suggested to account for at least some of the rapid increases in the rates of obesity, type II diabetes and cardiovascular disease recently observed in both developed and developing countries. This chapter will therefore focus on how nutritional cues in the environment can alter the epigenome, producing different phenotypes and altered disease susceptibilities from a single genotype.

Keywords: Epigenetics, nutrition, early life environment, DNA methylation, obesity, PPARS, adult onset disease, demethylases, transgenerational transmission developmental plasticity, mismatch.

5.1. EARLY LIFE ENVIRONMENT AND FUTURE DISEASE RISK

The association between the quality of early life environment and the subsequent risk of chronic disease in later life was first described in a series of epidemiological studies by David Barker and colleagues in the UK (1986). They found a strong geographical relationship between infant mortality and risk of cardiovascular disease (CVD) 50-60 years later [1]. Subsequent retrospective studies in cohorts across the globe in developed and developing nations including

*Address correspondence to Karen A. Lillycrop: Institute of Developmental Sciences, Mailpoint 887, Southampton General Hospital, Tremona Road, Southampton So16 6YD, UK; Phone: 44 2380 798663; Fax: 442380 798079; Email: kal@soton.ac.uk

Marcelina Párrizas, Rosa Gasa and Perla Kaliman (Eds)

the UK, North America, India and China [2] have shown consistently that lower birth weight within the normal range for a particular population is associated with an increased risk in later life of CVD and the metabolic syndrome (hypertension, insulin resistance, type 2 diabetes, dyslipidaemia and obesity) [2]. At the highest birth weight, the risk of disease again increases, resulting in a U- or J-shaped relationship between birth weight and later disease risk [3, 4]. However, birth weight in all of these studies should be viewed only as a very crude indicator of the intrauterine environment, which may have been compromised through a variety of maternal, environmental or placental factors [5]. And there is growing awareness that the factors which compromise foetal growth or nutrition need not be severe; for example, foetal growth is known to be constrained in those who are born to smaller mothers, in primigravida or in very young mothers [6].

The role of maternal diet on subsequent disease susceptibility has however been most clearly shown in studies of the Dutch Hunger Winter, a famine which occurred in the Netherlands during the winter of 1944. These studies have shown that individuals whose mothers were exposed to famine periconceptually and in the first trimester of pregnancy did not have reduced birth weights as compared to unexposed individuals, but as adults exhibited an increased risk of obesity and CVD, whereas individuals whose mothers were exposed in the later stages of gestation had reduced birth weights and showed increased incidence of insulin resistance and hypertension [7]. These studies suggest that the timing of the nutritional constraint during pregnancy is also important in determining the future risk of disease.

Early catch-up growth in infants born pre-term and fed formula milk is also related to increased risk of cardio-metabolic disease, including obesity, in later life [8-10]. A number of studies have shown a greater incidence of obesity in adults who were formula-fed as opposed to breast-fed during infancy [10, 11], although not all studies have found this [12]. An adequate fat mass is important for the onset of reproductive function, particularly in females [13]. In an evolutionary context, it is logical that catch-up growth in children born with a lower birth weight is characterized by greater adiposity relative to lean body mass, possibly as a mechanism to reach puberty at a similar age to peers born at greater weights. Although obesity is a risk factor for CVD, it has little negative effect in terms of potential reproductive success and so the trade-off associated with this strategy in terms of fitness is small.

Overnutrition in early life is also associated with an increased susceptibility to metabolic disease, which may account for the U-shaped or J-shaped relationships observed between birth weight and risk of obesity or insulin resistance in later life. Dorner and Plagemann (1994) have reported that children of obese women are themselves more likely to become overweight and develop insulin resistance in later life [14]. Gestational weight gain irrespective of pre-pregnancy weight is positively associated with obesity at 3 years old [15], and even moderate weight gain between successive pregnancies has been shown to result in a significant increase in large for gestational age (LGA) births [16]. However, maternal weight loss through bariatric surgery prevents transmission of obesity to children compared with the offspring of mothers who did not undergo the surgery and remained obese [17].

5.2. ANIMAL MODELS OF NUTRITIONAL PROGRAMMING

The first demonstration that unbalanced maternal nutrition can increase susceptibility to disease in later life in the offspring was made by Winick and Noble (1996), who showed that undernutrition during pregnancy in rats led to a reduced cell number in a range of tissues including the pancreas [18]. Subsequently, many groups have used sheep or rodents fed an isocaloric low protein diet, global dietary restriction or a high-fat diet during pregnancy and/or lactation to investigate the mechanisms by which nutrition in early life can influence development and alter later susceptibility to disease. Interestingly, offspring born to dams fed these different diets exhibit, to varying extents, characteristics of humans with cardio-metabolic disease including obesity, insulin resistance, hypertension and raised serum cholesterol levels. Together, these studies support the hypothesis that nutritional imbalance during prenatal and early postnatal life can induce long-term metabolic changes and increased susceptibility to metabolic disease in later life.

5.2.1. The Maternal Protein-Restricted Diet

The best-studied and most characterised animal model of nutritional induction of an altered phenotype is feeding pregnant rodents a protein-restricted (PR) diet.

Feeding a PR diet during pregnancy has been reported to result in impaired glucose homeostasis [19], vascular dysfunction [20], impaired immunity [21], increased susceptibility to oxidative stress [22], increased fat deposition and altered feeding behaviour [23, 24]. The induction during early life of persistent changes to the phenotype of the offspring by perturbations of the maternal diet implies stable alteration of gene transcription which in turn results in the altered activities of metabolic pathways and homeostatic control processes. Initially, using a candidate gene approach, many groups reported long-term changes in the expression of key metabolic genes in response to variations in maternal diet. For example, feeding a PR diet to pregnant rats increased glucocorticoid receptor (NR3C1) expression and reduced expression of 11β-hydroxysteroid dehydrogenase type II (*hsd11b2*), the enzyme that inactivates corticosteroids, in liver, lung, kidney and brain of the offspring [25]. In the liver, increased GR activity up-regulates phosphoenolpyruvate carboxykinase (*pepck*) expression and activity, thus increasing the capacity for gluconeogenesis. This may contribute to the induction of insulin resistance in this model [26]. Altered expression of *gr* has also been reported in the lung, liver, adrenal gland and kidney of the offspring of sheep fed a restricted diet during pregnancy [27-29]. Feeding a PR diet to pregnant rats up-regulates glucokinase (*gck*) expression in the liver of the offspring which implies increased capacity for glucose uptake [30]. The expression of genes involved in lipid homeostasis is also altered by maternal PR. Peroxisomal proliferator-activated receptor alpha (*ppara*) expression was increased in the liver of the offspring of rats fed a PR diet during pregnancy and was accompanied by up-regulation of its target gene acyl-Coenzyme A oxidase (*acox1*) [31]. The expression of acetyl-CoA carboxylase and fatty acid synthase (*fasn*) have also been reported to be increased in the liver of the offspring of rats fed a PR diet during pregnancy and lactation [32].

More recently, however, genome-wide approaches have been used to determine which genes are altered in response to diet. The transcriptome analysis of adult liver from PR offspring revealed that approximately 1.3% of genes within the genome is changed in response to maternal PR. The change in a relatively small subset of genes suggests that these may represent an orchestrated response to the nutritional challenge and be part of an adaptive response [33]. The pathways changed in the liver in response to maternal PR were developmental process, ion transport, response to hormone and response to stress, which is consistent with the phenotypic changes observed in PR offspring.

The alterations to the metabolism and physiology of the offspring induced by maternal protein restriction are dependent upon the timing of the nutritional challenge. Bertram *et al.* (2008) have shown in the guinea pig model that female offspring born to dams fed a PR diet in the first half of pregnancy (1-35 days) have raised mean arterial blood pressure associated with increased intraventricular septum (IVS) and anterior left ventricle wall (LVW) thickness. However, they did not exhibit growth restriction at any time. In contrast, the offspring from dams fed a PR diet in late gestation (36-70 days) were growth restricted but did not display alterations in blood pressure or LV structure [34].

Animal studies have also shown a clear interaction between prenatal and postnatal environments [35, 36]. For example, even modest variations in the diet fed after weaning can exacerbate the effects of maternal undernutrition on the phenotype of the offspring. Dyslipidaemia and impaired glucose homeostasis induced by feeding dams a PR diet during pregnancy were exacerbated in adult male and female rats fed a diet containing 10% (w/w) fat after weaning compared to a 4% (w/w) fat post-weaning diet [37].

5.2.2. Global Dietary Restriction

A number of groups have also used global dietary restriction during pregnancy to investigate how maternal diet can influence disease susceptibility in later life. Woodall and co-workers (1996) used a global nutrient restriction of 30% of an *ad libitum* diet throughout gestation that results in a rat model of intrauterine growth retardation [38]. Offspring born to dams fed this diet during pregnancy are significantly smaller at birth than control offspring. They also exhibit higher systolic blood pressure, hyperinsulinaemia, hyperleptinaemia, hyperphagia, reduced locomotion and obesity. These metabolic alterations are all augmented by feeding a high-fat postnatal diet [39]. However, even modest global nutrient restriction during pregnancy has been shown to induce alterations in metabolism and the HPA axis. In guinea pigs fed an 85% of an *ad libitum* diet throughout gestation, alterations in postnatal cholesterol homeostasis were observed in the male offspring [40]. In the sheep, a 15% global nutrient restriction during the first half of pregnancy led to reduced adrenocorticotropic hormone (ACTH) and cortisol responses to exogenous corticotropin-releasing hormone and arginine vasopressin administration, and also a blunted cortisol response to ACTH [41]. Long-term changes in gene expression have also been reported in adult offspring of dams fed a global undernutrition diet during pregnancy. Gluckman *et al.* (2007) have shown that expression of *ppara* and *gr* are both down-regulated in adult offspring born to dams fed a global nutrient-restricted diet of 30% *ad libitum* during pregnancy [42].

5.2.3. High-fat Diet During Pregnancy

With recent concerns about the levels of obesity in the western world, a number of new animal models of overnutrition during pregnancy have also been developed. Feeding an obesogenic diet to female rats from before mating and through lactation has been shown to lead to maternal obesity as well as hyperphagia, increased adiposity, decreased muscle mass, reduced locomotive activity and accelerated puberty in the offspring [43]. Samuelsson *et al.* (2008) have also shown that offspring from pregnant rats fed a 'junk food diet' of 16% fat and 33% sugar throughout pregnancy and lactation exhibited higher blood pressure, greater adiposity and insulin resistance in comparison to control offspring [44]. The type of fat, however, may also be important, as dams fed diets high in essential fatty acids throughout late gestation and lactation produce offspring which eat less, are leaner and have improved insulin sensitivity as adults [45]. High-carbohydrate diets are also protective and produce offspring that remain lighter in weight [46]. Persistent alterations in the expression of *pparg2*, *hsd11b1* and the β2 and β3 adrenoreceptors in adipose tissue [44], which may lead to increased adipogenesis and decreased lipolysis, were also seen in these rats. Interestingly, studies by Ng *et al.* (2010) have shown that not only can variations in maternal diet affect subsequent phenotype but also that paternal diet is important in determining future disease risk. Paternal high-fat diet (HFD) exposure induces increased body weight, adiposity, impaired glucose tolerance and insulin sensitivity in female offspring [47]. Paternal HFD altered the expression of 642 pancreatic islet genes in adult female offspring; these genes included those involved in cation and ATP binding, cytoskeleton and intracellular transport.

There is also increasing evidence that the period of susceptibility extends into postnatal life as the suckling period has been shown to be critical in the developmental induction of metabolic disease. Studies of rats in cross-fostering experiments show that high-fat feeding in the suckling period leads to an increase in adiposity, hyperleptinaemia, and hypertension in the adult offspring fed a normal diet after weaning [48-50]. Schmidt *et al.* (2001) have also shown that overfeeding rats during the suckling period by rearing them in small litters produces hyperphagia and obesity in adults [51]. There is growing evidence that overnutrition during prenatal and/or early postnatal life alters the maturation of the appetite- and energy-regulating neural network in the hypothalamus. Overfeeding rat pups by rearing them in small litters leads to increased food intake in the perinatal period and this was also associated with a persistent increase in appetite drive in later life [52, 53]. In rodents, exposure to a diabetic environment before birth or exposure in early postnatal life results in significant changes in the architecture of the hypothalamus and a reduced sensitivity of hypothalamic neuropeptides to signals of increased nutrition, as well as central resistance to peripheral signals of satiety [54-56]. The effect of overnutrition on hypothalamus function has been observed not only in rodents where appetite circuits are not fully mature until postnatal day 16 [53] but also in sheep, where the neural network is relatively mature at birth as is in humans [57].

5.3. DEVELOPMENTAL PLASTICITY

Taken together, human epidemiological data and animal studies demonstrate that the prenatal and early postnatal periods play a critical role in the induction of metabolic disease in later life. Gluckman and Hanson (2004) have suggested that the changes induced by maternal under- or overnutrition may reflect an adaptive response of the foetus to environmental cues acting through the process of developmental plasticity which allows an organism to adjust its developmental programme, resulting in long-term changes in its metabolism and physiology in order to be better adapted to the future environment [58]. For instance, poor maternal nutrition may signal to the foetus that nutrients are scarce and an uncertain life course lies ahead. The foetus may then adapt its metabolism to conserve energy demands, increase its propensity to store fat, accelerate puberty and invest less in bone and muscle mass. If nutrition is poor in the postnatal environment, then the metabolism of the organism will be matched to the environment and that individual would be of low disease risk. In support of this, there is evidence in both rat and pig models of maternal overnutrition during pregnancy that continued high-fat feeding in postnatal life does not lead to deleterious effects [59, 60]. However, if the offspring does not predict correctly the environment experienced after birth, then it is at increased risk of developing cardiovascular and metabolic disease because its metabolism and homeostatic capacity is mismatched to its environment. This mismatch pathway may explain why a nutritional constraint in early life followed by an adequate or nutritionally rich postnatal diet will result in a greater risk of metabolic compromise [61]. One important feature of such adaptive changes during development is that different phenotypes can be generated from a single genome depending on the environment that the organism experiences. There is now increasing evidence that the mechanism by which different phenotypes are generated from a single genome is through the altered epigenetic regulation of genes.

5.4. EPIGENETICS

Epigenetic processes are integral in determining when and where specific genes are expressed. Alterations in the epigenetic regulation of genes can lead therefore to profound changes in phenotype [62, 63]. The major epigenetic processes are DNA methylation, histone modification and microRNAs. To date, most studies of the effect of early life nutrition on the epigenetic regulation of genes have focused on DNA methylation.

Methylation at the 5' position of cytosine in DNA within a CpG dinucleotide (the p denotes the intervening phosphate group) is a common modification in mammalian genomes and constitutes a stable epigenetic mark that is transmitted through DNA replication and cell division [64]. CpG dinucleotides are not randomly distributed throughout the genome but are clustered at the 5' ends of genes/promoters in regions known as CpG islands. Hypermethylation of these CpG islands is associated with transcriptional repression, while hypomethylation of CpG islands is associated with transcriptional activation [63, 65, 66]. DNA methylation is largely established during early life and essentially maintained throughout life, although gradual hypomethylation does occur during aging and such age-related alterations in methylation have been linked with cancer [67]. However, environmental perturbations during periods when methylation patterns are being established may impair the programme of gene control with potential long-term adverse consequences.

5.4.1. Diet and Altered Epigenetic Regulation

One of the best examples of how diet can alter the phenotype and the importance of DNA methylation in phenotype induction is seen in the honeybee. Female larvae fed different diets develop into either sterile worker bees or fertile queen bees, even though they are genetically identical [68]. However, silencing the expression of DNA methyltransferase 3 (*dnmt3*) in pooled larvae increased the proportion of larvae developing into queen bees as opposed to sterile workers just as if the larvae had been fed royal jelly, suggesting that DNA methylation plays a key role in nutritional programming of the phenotype [68].

Alterations in DNA methylation have also been linked to nutritional programming of the phenotype in rodents. Differences in the intake of methyl donors and the cofactors for 1-carbon metabolism during pregnancy in the agouti mouse induce differences in the coat colour of the offspring. The murine A^{vy} mutation results from the insertion of an intracisternal-A particle (IAP) retrotransposon upstream of the agouti gene, which regulates the production of yellow-pigmented fur. This IAP acts as a cryptic promoter directing the expression of the agouti gene. Supplementation of pregnant mice with betaine, choline, folic acid and vitamin B_{12} shifted the distribution of coat colour of the offspring from yellow (agouti) to brown (pseudo-agouti) [69]. This shift is due to increased methylation of seven CpG dinucleotides located 600 bp downstream of the A^{vy} IAP insertion site.

Feeding pregnant rats a PR diet induced hypomethylation of the *gr* and *ppara* promoters in the livers of juvenile and adult offspring, and this was associated with increased mRNA expression of these genes (Fig. **1**) [31, 70]. This was the first evidence that moderate changes in macronutrient intake during pregnancy can alter the epigenome. Increased expression was associated with an increase in transcription-facilitating histone modifications at the *gr* promoter, in particular acetylation of histones H3 and H4 and methylation of histone H3 at lysine K4 (H3K4me), while those that suppress gene expression were reduced or unchanged

[71]. Altered methylation status of the liver *ppara* promoter was due to hypomethylation of four specific CpG dinucleotides, two of which predicted the level of the mRNA transcript, in juvenile offspring which persisted in adults [72]. Because the altered CpGs corresponded to transcription factor binding sites, this suggests a mechanism by which changes in the epigenetic regulation of genes established during development determine stimulus-specific responses in transcription, and thus the capacity of the tissue to face metabolic challenge. The angiotensin receptor 1b promoter is also hypomethylated in adrenal glands from PR offspring [73].

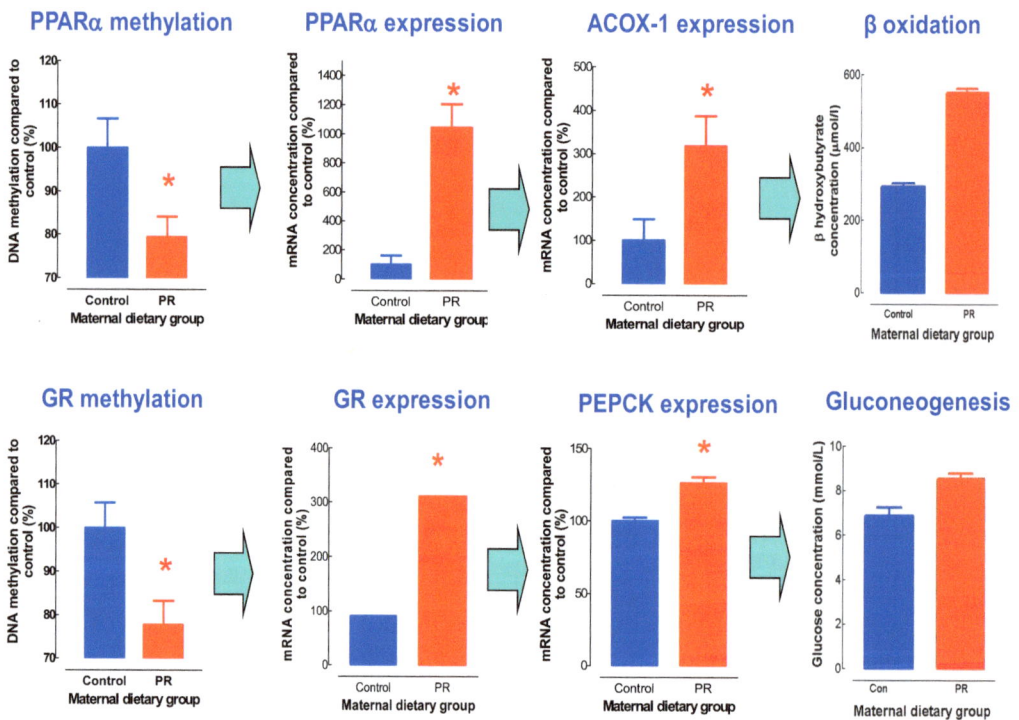

Figure 1: Maternal protein restriction induces altered methylation of the promoter regions of PPARα and GR in the liver of adult offspring from control and PR dams. Altered methylation is accompanied by an increase in the expression of *ppara* and *gr*, their target genes acetyl-CoA oxidase (*acox1*) and phosphoenolpyruvate carboxykinase (*pepck*), and the metabolic processes that they control, namely β oxidation and gluconeogenesis respectively.

Maternal global undernutrition also induces a phenotype in the offspring that resembles human metabolic syndrome [39]. In contrast to the effect of the maternal PR diet, adult female offspring of dams which experienced 70%

reduction in total nutrient intake during pregnancy showed hypermethylation and decreased expression of the *gr* and *ppara* promoters in the liver [42]. Thus, the effects of maternal nutrition on the epigenome of the offspring depend upon the nature of the maternal nutrient challenge.

There is also evidence that an overly rich early nutritional environment can alter the epigenetic regulation of genes. Plagemann *et al.* (2009) showed that neonatal overfeeding induced by raising rat pups in small litters induces the hypermethylation of two CpG dinucleotides within the pro-opiomelanocortin (*pomc*) promoter that are essential for *pomc* induction by leptin and insulin. Consequently, *pomc* expression is not up-regulated in these rats despite hyperinsulinaemia and hyperleptinaemia [74]. This suggests that overfeeding during early postnatal life, when the appetite circuitry within the hypothalamus is still developing, can alter the methylation of genes critical for body weight regulation, resulting in the altered programming of this system and an increased tendency towards obesity in later life. Ng *et al.* (2010) have also shown that the interleukin 13 receptor alpha 2 (*Il13ra2*) promoter was hypomethylated in female offspring after high-fat feeding of the fathers [47].

5.4.2. Evidence from Human Studies of Induced Epigenetic Change by Maternal Nutrition

In humans, Heijmans *et al.* (2008) have reported hypomethylation of the imprinted insulin-like growth factor-2 (*IGF2*) gene in genomic DNA isolated from whole blood cells from individuals who were exposed to famine *in utero* during the Dutch Hunger Winter compared to unexposed same-sex siblings [75]. The same group also found that *IGF2* was hypomethylated in individuals whose mothers were peri-conceptually exposed to famine, while *IL10*, leptin, ATP binding cassette A1 (*ABCA1*) and the paternally expressed antisense transcript of the stimulatory G protein alpha subunit (*GNASAS*) were hypermethylated [76]. The maximum difference between exposed and unexposed individuals was 6%. Although statistically significant, such small differences are difficult to interpret but do suggest that early life nutritional environment may induce persistent changes in the methylation of key regulatory genes in humans as in rodents.

5.4.3. Transgenerational Transmission of Altered Epigenetic Gene Regulation

Human studies have provided evidence for non-genomic transmission between generations of induced phenotypic traits associated with impaired metabolic homeostasis [77, 78]. Feeding a PR diet to pregnant rats in the F_0 generation resulted in elevated blood pressure and endothelial dysfunction [79] in both the F_1 and F_2 generations, despite normal nutrition during pregnancy in the F_1 generation. Hypomethylation of the hepatic *gr* and *ppara* promoters was also observed in both the F_1 and F_2 male offspring [70], suggesting that transmission of a phenotype induced in the F_1 generation to the F_2 generation may be mediated through an epigenetic mechanism. The mechanism by which induced epigenetic marks are transmitted to subsequent generations however is not known. As the transmission in this case was only to the F_2 generation, a direct effect of the diet given to the F_0 dams on the germ cells that gave rise to the F_2 offspring cannot be excluded. Further experiments examining transmission from F_1 to F_3, and further are required to determine the mechanism by which altered phenotype and epigenetic marks are transmitted from one generation to another.

5.4.4. Mechanisms for Induced Changes in the Epigenome

The mechanism by which nutrition in early life alters the epigenome is not known. *De novo* methylation of CpG dinucleotides is catalysed by DNA methyltransferases (DNMT) 3a and 3b, and is maintained through mitosis by gene-specific methylation of hemimethylated DNA by DNMT1 [64]. Although DNA methylation is regarded as a stable epigenetic mark, a number of DNA demethylases have been proposed, including MBD2 [80], MBD4 [81], the DNA repair endonucleases XPG (GADD45A) [82] and a G/T mismatch repair DNA glycosylase [83]. Although the evidence indicating that these particular proteins fulfil this role is at present very limited, there is clear proof that DNA demethylase activity exists in cells during development. Active demethylation has been observed on the paternal genomic DNA in the zygote upon fertilization [84], on the synaptic plasticity gene reelin in the hippocampus upon contextual fear conditioning [85] and on the interferon gamma (*ifng*) gene upon antigen exposure of memory CD8 T cells [86]. Syzf (2007) has also proposed that the methylation status of CpGs in post-mitotic cells may represent an equilibrium state dependent upon the relative activities of DNMT1 and demethylases [87]. Thus, environmental exposures, which alter the activity of the DNMTs and/or demethylases, provide a possible mechanism by which a change in methylation could occur.

Feeding a PR diet to rats during pregnancy decreased the expression of *dnmt1*, but not that of *dnmt3a* and *dnmt3b* which regulate *de novo* DNA methylation [71]. This suggests that hypomethylation of the *gr* and *ppara* promoters in the liver of the offspring may be caused by a failure to maintain methylation patterns during mitosis [71, 88]. This is supported by the finding that the decrease in *dnmt1* expression observed in the offspring of dams fed a PR diet was prevented by increasing the folic acid content of the PR diet [71]. Reduced DNMT1 activity might be expected to result in global DNA demethylation; however, a decrease in *dnmt1* expression has been reported to result only in a subset of genes being demethylated [89], suggesting that DNMT1 is targeted to specific genes. Accordingly, several reports have shown that DNMT1 interacts with a number of histone modifying enzymes and is targeted to specific DNA sites [90-92]. Interestingly, hyperglycaemia and hyperinsulinaemia have been reported to favour homocysteine remethylation, leading to increased intracellular concentrations of S-adenosyl methionine and enhanced DNA methyltransferase activity [93], supporting findings from previous undernutrition studies that the methylation balance and regulation of DNA methyltransferases are sensitive to nutritional environmental cues (Fig. **2**).

5.4.5. Prevention and Reversal of an Altered Phenotype and Epigenotype

A number of studies have shown that, despite the apparent stability of methylation marks, alterations in DNA methylation induced by maternal diet can be prevented and even reversed by interventions in postnatal life. Supplementation of the maternal PR diet with folic acid prevents hypertension, vascular dysfunction and dyslipidaemia in the adult offspring [94]. Increasing the folic acid content of the PR diet also prevented the hypomethylation of the *ppara* and *gr* promoters and restored levels of GR and PPARα expression to those seen in control offspring. As mentioned before, folic acid supplementation of PR diet during pregnancy also up-regulated *dnmt1* expression [31]. This suggests that impaired 1-carbon metabolism plays a central role in the establishment of the altered epigenetic regulation of *gr* and *ppara* and the development of an altered phenotype by maternal protein restriction. Interestingly, detailed analysis of the *ppara* promoter showed that although increased maternal folic acid intake prevented hypomethylation of the majority of CpG dinucleotides induced by the PR diet alone, two CpGs were hypermethylated [72]. Thus, increasing maternal folic acid intake does not simply prevent the effects of the PR diet, but may induce subtle changes in gene regulation. Burdge *et al.* (2009) have also shown that folate supplementation during the juvenile-pubertal period altered both the phenotype and epigenotype induced by a maternal PR diet [95]. These results showed that in contrast to supplementation of the maternal PR diet with folic acid, supplementation during the juvenile-pubertal period caused impaired lipid homeostasis including down-regulation of hepatic fatty acid β-oxidation, hepatic steatosis and increased weight gain, irrespective of the maternal diet. This was associated with altered methylation of specific genes, including hypermethylation of *ppara* in the liver and hypomethylation of the insulin receptor in adipose tissue. These findings suggest that in rats the period between weaning and adulthood represents a period of increased plasticity, where it may be possible to reverse adverse effect of prenatal nutrition by interventions.

Supplementation of the maternal diet with methyl donors also prevented the transgenerational amplification of obesity observed in A^{vy} mice [96], supporting the hypothesis that altered epigenetic regulation underlies the mechanism by which maternal obesity increases susceptibility of their offspring to obesity in later life. The effect of methyl supplementation on body weight was independent of epigenetic changes at the A^{vy} locus, suggesting that maternal obesity alters the methylation at other sites in the genome, potentially genes involved in appetite and energy balance, and that methyl supplementation blocks such epigenetic dysregulation.

Treatment with leptin between postnatal days 3 and 13 of neonatal rats born to dams which experienced 70% global reduction in food intake during pregnancy normalised caloric intake, locomotive activity, body weight, fat mass and fasting plasma glucose, insulin and leptin concentrations in adult offspring in contrast to saline treated offspring of undernourished dams who developed all these features on a high-fat diet [97]. This again shows that developmental metabolic programming is potentially reversible by an intervention late in the phase of developmental plasticity. The ability of leptin to reverse these metabolic effects has been suggested to occur as a result of leptin administration giving a false developmental cue signalling adiposity to the pups that were actually thin and thus setting their metabolic phenotype to be more appropriate to a high nutrition environment. Strikingly, the corrective effects of leptin were paralleled by effects on methylation and expression of *ppara* and *gr* [42]. This suggests that neonatal leptin intervention may exert its corrective adaptive effects through epigenetic mechanisms.

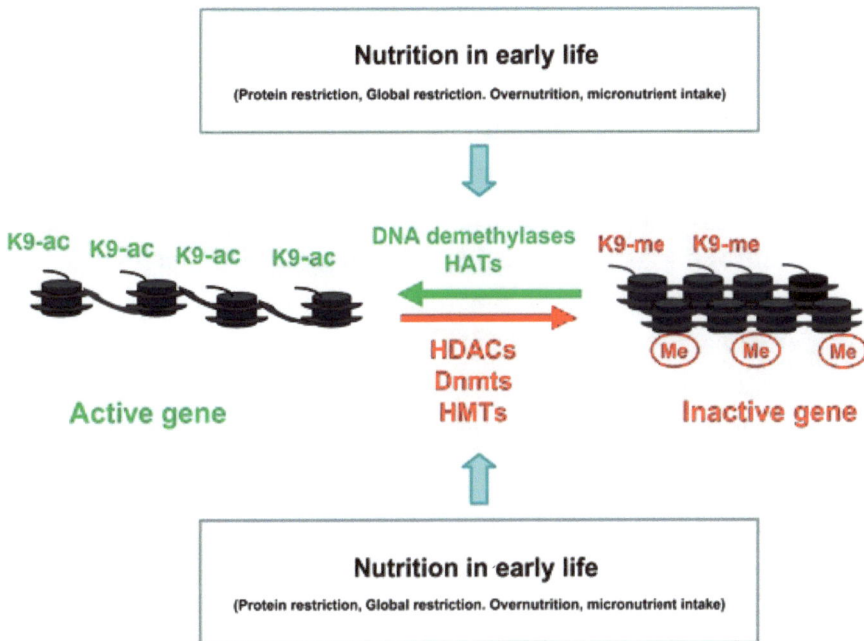

Figure 2: Effect of early life nutrition on the epigenome. Nutrition in early life determines the balance between gene methylation and demethylation. Histone deacetylases (HDACs), histone methyltransferases (HMTs) and DNA methyltransferases (DNMTs) promote histone deacetylation, histone H3K9 methylation and DNA methylation, resulting in a closed chromatin configuration and gene silencing. Histone acetyltransferases (HATs) and DNA demethylases induce histone acetylation and DNA demethylation resulting in an open chromatin configuration and gene transcription.

CONCLUSIONS

Traditionally, DNA sequence was believed to be the sole determinant of phenotype, and phenotypic variation was considered to be a result of genetic mutation or recombination. There is now evidence that epigenetic mechanisms allow the developing foetus to adapt to nutritional cues from the mother and adjust its developmental trajectory to produce a phenotype matched to the predicted postnatal environment. Studies from both animal models and humans suggest that altered epigenetic marks induced by early environmental challenges are stably maintained throughout the life course raising the possibility that these altered marks may be used as predictive markers of later phenotype and disease risk. Animal studies also suggest that these altered epigenetic marks can be prevented and/or reversed at specific time periods, implying that it may be possible either through nutritional or pharmaceutical interventions to reverse such epigenetic marks and reduce the incidence of non-communicable diseases. However there is still much we have to understand. For instance, what early life exposures can alter the epigenome? How are environmental signals transmitted from mother to foetus? What are the critical developmental periods? Do these differ depending on the tissue? And can interventions be targeted to specific epigenetic marks? With this increased level of understanding of the relationship between epigenetics, the environment and disease susceptibility it may then be possible to make real progress in the prevention and treatment of chronic diseases and halt the rapid rise in non-communicable diseases currently seen throughout the world.

DISCLOSURE

"Part of information included in this chapter has been previously published in International Journal of Obesity (2011) 35, 72–83".

REFERENCES

[1]   Barker DJ, Osmond C. Infant mortality, childhood nutrition, and ischaemic heart disease in England and Wales. Lancet 1986; 1: 1077-81.
[2]   Godfrey KM, Barker DJ. Fetal programming and adult health. Public Health Nutr 2001; 4: 611-24.
[3]   Curhan GC, Willett WC, Rimm EB, Spiegelman D, Ascherio AL, Stampfer MJ. Birth weight and adult hypertension, diabetes mellitus, and obesity in US men. Circulation 1996; 94: 3246-50.

[4]   McCance DR, Pettitt DJ, Hanson RL, Jacobsson LT, Knowler WC, Bennett PH. Birth weight and non-insulin dependent diabetes: thrifty genotype, thrifty phenotype, or surviving small baby genotype? BMJ 1994; 308: 942-5.

[5]   Hanson MA, Gluckman PD. Developmental processes and the induction of cardiovascular function: conceptual aspects. J Physiol 2005; 565(Pt 1): 27-34.

[6]   Gluckman PD, Hanson MA. Developmental and epigenetic pathways to obesity: an evolutionary-developmental perspective. Int J Obes (Lond) 2008; 32(Suppl 7): S62-S71.

[7]   Painter RC, Roseboom TJ, Bleker OP. Prenatal exposure to the Dutch famine and disease in later life: an overview. Reprod Toxicol 2005; 20: 345-52.

[8]   Singhal A, Cole TJ, Fewtrell M, Lucas A. Breastmilk feeding and lipoprotein profile in adolescents born preterm: follow-up of a prospective randomised study. Lancet 2004; 363: 1571-8.

[9]   Singhal A. Early nutrition and long-term cardiovascular health. Nutr Rev 2006; 64(5 Pt 2): S44-S49.

[10]   Harder T, Bergmann R, Kallischnigg G, Plagemann A. Duration of breastfeeding and risk of overweight: a meta-analysis. Am J Epidemiol 2005; 162: 397-403.

[11]   Owen CG, Martin RM, Whincup PH, Smith GD, Cook DG. Effect of infant feeding on the risk of obesity across the life course: a quantitative review of published evidence. Pediatrics 2005; 115: 1367-77.

[12]   Owen CG, Martin RM, Whincup PH, Davey-Smith G, Gillman MW, Cook DG. The effect of breastfeeding on mean body mass index throughout life: a quantitative review of published and unpublished observational evidence. Am J Clin Nutr 2005; 82: 1298-307.

[13]   Gluckman PD, Hanson MA. Evolution, development and timing of puberty. Trends Endocrinol Metab 2006; 17: 7-12.

[14]   Dorner G, Plagemann A. Perinatal hyperinsulinism as possible predisposing factor for diabetes mellitus, obesity and enhanced cardiovascular risk in later life. Horm Metab Res 1994; 26: 213-21.

[15]   Oken E, Taveras EM, Kleinman KP, Rich-Edwards JW, Gillman MW. Gestational weight gain and child adiposity at age 3 years. Am J Obstet Gynecol 2007; 196: 322-8.

[16]   Villamor E, Cnattingius S. Interpregnancy weight change and risk of adverse pregnancy outcomes: a population-based study. Lancet 2006; 368: 1164-70.

[17]   Kral JG, Biron S, Simard S, Hould FS, Lebel S, Marceau S, *et al.* Large maternal weight loss from obesity surgery prevents transmission of obesity to children who were followed for 2 to 18 years. Pediatrics 2006; 118: e1644-9.

[18]   Winick M, Noble A. Cellular response in rats during malnutrition at various ages. J Nutr 1966; 89: 300-6.

[19]   Fernandez-Twinn DS, Wayman A, Ekizoglou S, Martin MS, Hales CN, Ozanne SE. Maternal protein restriction leads to hyperinsulinemia and reduced insulin-signaling protein expression in 21-mo-old female rat offspring. Am J Physiol Regul Integr Comp Physiol 2005; 288: R368-73.

[20]   Torrens C, Brawley L, Anthony FW, Dance CS, Dunn R, Jackson AA, *et al.* Folate supplementation during pregnancy improves offspring cardiovascular dysfunction induced by protein restriction. Hypertension 2006; 47: 982-7.

[21]   Calder PC, Yaqoob P. The level of protein and type of fat in the diet of pregnant rats both affect lymphocyte function in the offspring. Nutr Res 2000; 20: 995-1005.

[22]   Langley-Evans SC, Sculley DV. Programming of hepatic antioxidant capacity and oxidative injury in the ageing rat. Mech Ageing Dev 2005; 126: 804-12.

[23] Bellinger L, Lilley C, Langley-Evans SC. Prenatal exposure to a maternal low-protein diet programmes a preference for high-fat foods in the young adult rat. Br J Nutr 2004; 92: 513-20.

[24] Bellinger L, Sculley DV, Langley-Evans SC. Exposure to undernutrition in fetal life determines fat distribution, locomotor activity and food intake in ageing rats. Int J Obes (Lond) 2006; 30: 729-38.

[25] Bertram CE, Hanson MA. Animal models and programming of the metabolic syndrome. Br Med Bull 2001; 60: 103-21.

[26] Burns SP, Desai M, Cohen RD, Hales CN, Iles RA, Germain JP, *et al.* Gluconeogenesis, Glucose Handling, and Structural Changes in Livers of the Adult Offspring of Rats Partially Deprived of Protein During Pregnancy and Lactation. J Clin Invest 1997; 100: 1768-74.

[27] Whorwood CB, Firth KM, Budge H, Symonds ME. Maternal undernutrition during early to midgestation programs tissue-specific alterations in the expression of the glucocorticoid receptor, 11beta-hydroxysteroid dehydrogenase isoforms, and type 1 angiotensin II receptor in neonatal sheep. Endocrinology 2001; 142: 2854-64.

[28] Brennan KA, Gopalakrishnan GS, Kurlak L, Rhind SM, Kyle CE, Brooks AN, *et al.* Impact of maternal undernutrition and fetal number on glucocorticoid, growth hormone and insulin-like growth factor receptor mRNA abundance in the ovine fetal kidney. Reproduction 2005; 129: 151-9.

[29] Gnanalingham MG, Mostyn A, Dandrea J, Yakubu DP, Symonds ME, Stephenson T. Ontogeny and nutritional programming of uncoupling protein-2 and glucocorticoid receptor mRNA in the ovine lung. J Physiol 2005; 565(Pt 1): 159-69.

[30] Bogdarina I, Murphy HC, Burns SP, Clark AJ. Investigation of the role of epigenetic modification of the rat glucokinase gene in fetal programming. Life Sci 2004; 74: 1407-15.

[31] Lillycrop KA, Phillips ES, Jackson AA, Hanson MA, Burdge GC. Dietary protein restriction of pregnant rats induces and folic acid supplementation prevents epigenetic modification of hepatic gene expression in the offspring. J Nutr 2005; 135: 1382-6.

[32] Maloney CA, Gosby AK, Phuyal JL, Denyer GS, Bryson JM, Caterson ID. Site-specific changes in the expression of fat-partitioning genes in weanling rats exposed to a low-protein diet in utero. Obes Res 2003; 11: 461-8.

[33] Lillycrop KA, Rodford J, Garratt ES, Slater-Jefferies JL, Godfrey KM, Gluckman PD, *et al.* Maternal protein restriction with or without folic acid supplementation during pregnancy alters the hepatic transcriptome in adult male rats. Br J Nutr 2010; 103: 1711-9.

[34] Bertram C, Khan O, Ohri S, Phillips DI, Matthews SG, Hanson MA. Transgenerational effects of prenatal nutrient restriction on cardiovascular and hypothalamic-pituitary-adrenal function. J Physiol 2008; 586: 2217-29.

[35] Ozanne SE, Hales CN. Lifespan: catch-up growth and obesity in male mice. Nature 2004; 427: 411-2.

[36] Zambrano E, Bautista CJ, Deas M, Martinez-Samayoa PM, Gonzalez-Zamorano M, Ledesma H, *et al.* A low maternal protein diet during pregnancy and lactation has sex- and window of exposure-specific effects on offspring growth and food intake, glucose metabolism and serum leptin in the rat. J Physiol 2006; 571(Pt 1): 221-30.

[37] Burdge GC, Lillycrop KA, Jackson AA, Gluckman PD, Hanson MA. The nature of the growth pattern and of the metabolic response to fasting in the rat are dependent upon the dietary protein and folic acid intakes of their pregnant dams and post-weaning fat consumption. Br J Nutr 2008; 99: 540-9.

[38]   Woodall SM, Johnston BM, Breier BH, Gluckman PD. Chronic maternal undernutrition in the rat leads to delayed postnatal growth and elevated blood pressure of offspring. Pediatr Res 1996; 40: 438-43.

[39]   Vickers MH, Breier BH, Cutfield WS, Hofman PL, Gluckman PD. Fetal origins of hyperphagia, obesity, and hypertension and postnatal amplification by hypercaloric nutrition. Am J Physiol Endocrinol Metab 2000; 279: E83-7.

[40]   Kind KL, Clifton PM, Katsman AI, Tsiounis M, Robinson JS, Owens JA. Restricted]fetal growth and the response to dietary cholesterol in the guinea pig. Am J Physiol 1999; 277(6 Pt 2): R1675-82.

[41]   Hawkins P, Steyn C, McGarrigle HH, Saito T, Ozaki T, Stratford LL, *et al.* Effect of maternal nutrient restriction in early gestation on responses of the hypothalamic-pituitary-adrenal axis to acute isocapnic hypoxaemia in late gestation fetal sheep. Exp Physiol 2000; 85: 85-96.

[42]   Gluckman PD, Lillycrop KA, Vickers MH, Pleasants AB, Phillips ES, Beedle AS, *et al.* Metabolic plasticity during mammalian development is directionally dependent on early nutritional status. Proc Natl Acad Sci USA 2007; 104: 12796-800.

[43]   Guo F, Jen KL. High-fat feeding during pregnancy and lactation affects offspring metabolism in rats. Physiol Behav 1995; 57: 681-6.

[44]   Samuelsson AM, Matthews PA, Argenton M, Christie MR, McConnell JM, Jansen EH, *et al.* Diet-induced obesity in female mice leads to offspring hyperphagia, adiposity, hypertension, and insulin resistance: a novel murine model of developmental programming. Hypertension 2008; 51: 383-92.

[45]   Korotkova M, Gabrielsson BG, Holmang A, Larsson BM, Hanson LA, Strandvik B. Gender-related long-term effects in adult rats by perinatal dietary ratio of n-6/n-3 fatty acids. Am J Physiol Regul Integr Comp Physiol 2005; 288: R575-9.

[46]   Kozak R, Burlet A, Burlet C, Beck B. Dietary composition during fetal and neonatal life affects neuropeptide Y functioning in adult offspring. Brain Res Dev Brain Res 2000; 125: 75-82.

[47]   Ng SF, Lin RC, Laybutt DR, Barres R, Owens JA, Morris MJ. Chronic high-fat diet in fathers programs beta-cell dysfunction in female rat offspring. Nature 2010; 467: 963-6.

[48]   Khan IY, Dekou V, Douglas G, Jensen R, Hanson MA, Poston L, *et al.* A high-fat diet during rat pregnancy or suckling induces cardiovascular dysfunction in adult offspring. Am J Physiol Regul Integr Comp Physiol 2005; 288: R127-33.

[49]   Plagemann A, Harder T, Rake A, Melchior K, Rittel F, Rohde W, *et al.* Hypothalamic insulin and neuropeptide Y in the offspring of gestational diabetic mother rats. Neuroreport 1998; 9: 4069-73.

[50]   Plagemann A, Heidrich I, Gotz F, Rohde W, Dorner G. Obesity and enhanced diabetes and cardiovascular risk in adult rats due to early postnatal overfeeding. Exp Clin Endocrinol 1992; 99: 154-8.

[51]   Schmidt I, Fritz A, Scholch C, Schneider D, Simon E, Plagemann A. The effect of leptin treatment on the development of obesity in overfed suckling Wistar rats. Int J Obes Relat Metab Disord 2001; 25: 1168-74.

[52]   Davidowa H, Plagemann A. Decreased inhibition by leptin of hypothalamic arcuate neurons in neonatally overfed young rats. Neuroreport 2000; 11: 2795-8.

[53]   Plagemann A, Harder T, Rake A, Melchior K, Rohde W, Dorner G. Increased number of galanin-neurons in the paraventricular hypothalamic nucleus of neonatally overfed weanling rats. Brain Res 1999; 818: 160-3.

[54] Plagemann A, Harder T, Rake A, Melchior K, Rittel F, Rohde W, *et al.* Hypothalamic insulin and neuropeptide Y in the offspring of gestational diabetic mother rats. Neuroreport 1998; 9: 4069-73.

[55] Plagemann A, Harder T, Melchior K, Rake A, Rohde W, Dorner G. Elevation of hypothalamic neuropeptide Y-neurons in adult offspring of diabetic mother rats. Neuroreport 1999; 10: 3211-6.

[56] Plagemann A, Harder T, Janert U, Rake A, Rittel F, Rohde W, *et al.* Malformations of hypothalamic nuclei in hyperinsulinemic offspring of rats with gestational diabetes. Dev Neurosci 1999; 21: 58-67.

[57] Muhlhausler BS. Programming of the appetite-regulating neural network: a link between maternal overnutrition and the programming of obesity? J Neuroendocrinol 2007; 19: 67-72.

[58] Gluckman PD, Hanson MA. Developmental origins of disease paradigm: a mechanistic and evolutionary perspective. Pediatr Res 2004; 56: 311-7.

[59] Norman JF, LeVeen RF. Maternal atherogenic diet in swine is protective against early atherosclerosis development in offspring consuming an atherogenic diet post-natally. Atherosclerosis 2001; 157: 41-7.

[60] Khan I, Dekou V, Hanson M, Poston L, Taylor P. Predictive adaptive responses to maternal high-fat diet prevent endothelial dysfunction but not hypertension in adult rat offspring. Circulation 2004; 110: 1097-102.

[61] Gluckman PD, Hanson MA. The Fetal Matrix: Evolution, Developmental and Disease. Cambridge University Press; 2005.

[62] Cox GF, Burger J, Lip V, Mau UA, Sperling K, Wu BL, *et al.* Intracytoplasmic sperm]injection may increase the risk of imprinting defects. Am J Hum Genet 2002; 71: 162-4.

[63] DeBaun MR, Niemitz EL, Feinberg AP. Association of *in vitro* fertilization with Beckwith-Wiedemann syndrome and epigenetic alterations of LIT1 and H19. Am J Hum Genet 2003; 72: 156-60.

[64] Bird A. DNA methylation patterns and epigenetic memory. Genes Dev 2002; 16: 6-21.

[65] Bird AP. CpG-rich islands and the function of DNA methylation. Nature 1986; 21: 209-13.

[66] Reik W, Dean W. DNA methylation and mammalian epigenetics. Electrophoresis 2001; 22: 2838-43.

[67] Gonzalo S. Epigenetic alterations in aging. J Appl Physiol 2010; 109: 586-97.

[68] Kucharski R, Maleszka J, Foret S, Maleszka R. Nutritional control of reproductive status in honeybees *via* DNA methylation. Science 2008; 319: 1827-30.

[69] Wolff GL, Kodell RL, Moore SR, Cooney CA. Maternal epigenetics and methyl supplements affect agouti gene expression in Avy/a mice. FASEB J 1998; 12: 949-57.

[70] Burdge GC, Slater-Jefferies J, Torrens C, Phillips ES, Hanson MA, Lillycrop KA. Dietary protein restriction of pregnant rats in the F0 generation induces altered methylation of hepatic gene promoters in the adult male offspring in the F1 and F2 generations. Br J Nutr 2007; 97: 435-9.

[71] Lillycrop KA, Slater-Jefferies JL, Hanson MA, Godfrey KM, Jackson AA, Burdge GC. Induction of altered epigenetic regulation of the hepatic glucocorticoid receptor in the offspring of rats fed a protein-restricted diet during pregnancy suggests that reduced DNA methyltransferase-1 expression is involved in impaired DNA methylation and changes in histone modifications. Br J Nutr 2007; 97: 1064-73.

[72]   Lillycrop KA, Phillips ES, Torrens C, Hanson MA, Jackson AA, Burdge GC. Feeding pregnant rats a protein-restricted diet persistently alters the methylation of specific cytosines in the hepatic PPARalpha promoter of the offspring. Br J Nutr 2008; 100: 278-82.

[73]   Bogdarina I, Welham S, King PJ, Burns SP, Clark AJ. Epigenetic modification of the renin-angiotensin system in the fetal programming of hypertension. Circ Res 2007; 100: 520-6.

[74]   Plagemann A, Harder T, Brunn M, Harder A, Roepke K, Wittrock-Staar M, *et al.* Hypothalamic proopiomelanocortin promoter methylation becomes altered by early overfeeding: an epigenetic model of obesity and the metabolic syndrome. J Physiol 2009; 587(Pt 20): 4963-76.

[75]   Heijmans BT, Tobi EW, Stein AD, Putter H, Blauw GJ, Susser ES, *et al.* Persistent epigenetic differences associated with prenatal exposure to famine in humans. Proc Natl Acad Sci USA 2008; 105: 17046-9.

[76]   Tobi EW, Lumey LH, Talens RP, Kremer D, Putter H, Stein AD, *et al.* DNA methylation differences after exposure to prenatal famine are common and timing- and sex-specific. Hum Mol Genet 2009; 18: 4046-53.

[77]   Pembrey ME, Bygren LO, Kaati G, Edvinsson S, Northstone K, Sjostrom M, *et al.* Sex-specific, male-line transgenerational responses in humans. Eur J Hum Genet 2006; 14: 159-66.

[78]   Stein AD, Lumey LH. The relationship between maternal and offspring birth weights after maternal prenatal famine exposure: the Dutch Famine Birth Cohort Study. Hum Biol 2000; 72: 641-54.

[79]   Torrens C, Brawley L, Barker AC, Itoh S, Poston L, Hanson MA. Maternal protein restriction in the rat impairs resistance artery but not conduit artery function in pregnant offspring. J Physiol 2003; 547(Pt 1): 77-84.

[80]   Bhattacharya SK, Ramchandani S, Cervoni N, Szyf M. A mammalian protein with specific demethylase activity for mCpG DNA. Nature 1999; 397: 579-83.

[81]   Zhu B, Zheng Y, Hess D, Angliker H, Schwarz S, Siegmann M, *et al.* 5-methylcytosine-DNA glycosylase activity is present in a cloned G/T mismatch DNA glycosylase associated with the chicken embryo DNA demethylation complex. Proc Natl Acad Sci USA 2000; 97: 5135-9.

[82]   Barreto G, Schafer A, Marhold J, Stach D, Swaminathan SK, Handa V, *et al.* Gadd45a promotes epigenetic gene activation by repair-mediated DNA demethylation. Nature 2007; 445: 671-5.

[83]   Jost JP. Nuclear Extracts of Chicken Embryos Promote An Active Demethylation of Dna by Excision Repair of 5-Methyldeoxycytidine. Proc of the Natl Acad Sci USA 1993; 90: 4684-8.

[84]   Reik W, Dean W, Walter J. Epigenetic reprogramming in mammalian development. Science 2001; 293: 1089-93.

[85]   Miller CA, Sweatt JD. Covalent modification of DNA regulates memory formation. Neuron 2007; 53: 857-69.

[86]   Kersh EN, Fitzpatrick DR, Murali-Krishna K, Shires J, Speck SH, Boss JM, *et al.* Rapid demethylation of the IFN-gamma gene occurs in memory but not naive CD8 T cells. J Immunol 2006; 176: 4083-93.

[87]   Szyf M. The dynamic epigenome and its implications in toxicology. Toxicol Sci 2007; 100: 7-23.

[88]   Burdge GC, Hanson MA, Slater-Jefferies JL, Lillycrop KA. Epigenetic regulation of transcription: a mechanism for inducing variations in phenotype (fetal programming) by differences in nutrition during early life? Br J Nutr 2007; 97: 1036-46.

[89]   Jackson-Grusby L, Beard C, Possemato R, Tudor M, Fambrough D, Csankovszki G, *et al.* Loss of genomic methylation causes p53-dependent apoptosis and epigenetic deregulation. Nat Genet 2001; 27: 31-9.

[90]   Fuks F, Hurd PJ, Deplus R, Kouzarides T. The DNA methyltransferases associate with HP1 and the SUV39H1 histone methyltransferase. Nucleic Acids Res 2003; 31: 2305-12.

[91]   Rountree MR, Bachman KE, Baylin SB. DNMT1 binds HDAC2 and a new co-repressor, DMAP1, to form a complex at replication foci. Nat Genet 2000; 25: 269-77.

[92]   Vire E, Brenner C, Deplus R, Blanchon L, Fraga M, Didelot C, *et al.* The Polycomb group protein EZH2 directly controls DNA methylation. Nature 2006; 439: 871-4.

[93]   Chiang PK, Gordon RK, Tal J, Zeng GC, Doctor BP, Pardhasaradhi K, *et al.* S-Adenosylmethionine and methylation. FASEB J 1996; 10: 471-80.

[94]   Jackson AA, Dunn RL, Marchand MC, Langley-Evans SC. Increased systolic blood pressure in rats induced by a maternal low-protein diet is reversed by dietary supplementation with glycine. Clin Sci (Lond) 2002; 103: 633-9.

[95]   Burdge GC, Lillycrop KA, Phillips ES, Slater-Jefferies JL, Jackson AA, Hanson MA. Folic Acid Supplementation during the Juvenile-Pubertal Period in Rats Modifies the Phenotype and Epigenotype Induced by Prenatal Nutrition. J Nutr 2009; 139: 1054-60.

[96]   Waterland RA, Travisano M, Tahiliani KG, Rached MT, Mirza S. Methyl donor supplementation prevents transgenerational amplification of obesity. Int J Obes (Lond) 2008; 32: 1373-9.

[97]   Vickers MH, Gluckman PD, Coveny AH, Hofman PL, Cutfield WS, Gertler A, *et al.* Neonatal Leptin Treatment Reverses Developmental Programming. Endocrinology 2005; 146: 4211-6.

CHAPTER 6

Influences of Environmental Toxicants on the Human Epigenome

Jorge A. Alegría-Torres[1], Valentina Bollati[2] and Andrea Baccarelli[3,*]

[1]Departamento de Toxicologia Ambiental, Facultad de Medicina, Universidad Autonoma de San Luis Potosi, Mexico; [2]Center of Molecular and Genetic Epidemiology, Department of Environmental and Occupational Health, Università degli Studi di Milano and Fondazione IRCCS Ospedale Maggiore Policlinico, Mangiagalli e Regina Elena and [3]Exposure, Epidemiology and Risk Program, Department of Environmental Health, Harvard School of Public Health, Boston, Massachusetts, USA

Abstract: Epigenetics explores heritable changes in gene expression that occur without changes in DNA sequence. Several epigenetic mechanisms - among which DNA methylation, histone modifications and microRNA expression are the best studied - can adapt genome function to respond to environmental requirements. In this chapter, we review current evidences indicating that environmental agents are able to modify epigenetic markers. The epigenetic alterations induced by some exposures are the same as/or similar to epigenetic alterations found in patients with diseases. Several investigations have examined the relationship between exposure to environmental chemicals and epigenetics, and have identified toxicants that modify epigenetic states. Among these we will focus on exposure to particulate matter, heavy metals and organic compounds. We have also considered how the length of the exposure and the concentration of pollutants may modify the environment-epigenome interaction, and how genetic variability, prenatal exposure, and circadian rhythm may mitigate or overstate epigenetic disruptions.

Keywords: Epigenetic markers, environmental exposure, DNA methylation, histone modification, microRNA's, environment-epigenome interaction, particulate matters, heavy metals, organic compounds.

6.1. INTRODUCTION

According to the World Health Organization, a quarter of the diseases facing mankind today occur due to prolonged exposure to environmental pollution.

*****Address correspondence to Andrea Baccarelli:** Exposure, Epidemiology and Risk Program, Department of Environmental Health, Harvard School of Public Health, Boston, Massachusetts, USA; Phone: (617)384-8742; Fax: (617) 384-8859; Email: abaccare@hsph.harvard.edu

Because these toxicants are pervasive in our environment, are not usually measured for each person, and may produce effects even decades after the exposure, a major challenge in environmental health is to develop methods to identify individuals who are biologically damaged by their exposures, and to predict who will develop disease. In this context, epigenetics has received increasing consideration in environmental research as an untapped potential resource to identify mechanistic-based biomarkers of disease and exposure [1, 2].

Epigenetic mechanisms, including DNA methylation, histone modifications, and miRNAs, are flexible parameters that can change in response to environmental cues. The flexibility of epigenetic mechanisms has generated a growing interest in evaluating the alterations that environmental exposures may produce on epigenetic states, and whether such changes might activate pathways leading to detrimental effects on human health. These effects might be cumulative and take many years before any clinical manifestation is detected. Epigenetic mechanisms can be modified by the environment and such modifications might persist even in the absence of the factors that established them [3, 4]. Epigenetic changes have thus the potential to provide more stable biomarkers and fingerprints of exposure than those that have been developed from altered gene or protein expression [5]. In this review, we examine the evidence of environmental influences on epigenetics from experimental studies and epidemiological investigations (Table **1**).

6.2. PARTICULATE MATTER AIR POLLUTION

Human studies have shown that long-term exposure to air pollution, particularly to particulate matter, increases oxidative stress and inflammation [6-8], which in turn have been linked to morbidity and mortality from cardiorespiratory disease and lung cancer [9-13]. At a molecular level, exposure to particulate matter has been associated with accelerated biological aging, as reflected in the reduced telomere length in circulating blood leukocytes observed in a population of elderly smokers as well as in men exposed to traffic pollutants [14-16]. The G-rich structure of telomeres is highly sensitive to oxidative stress [14]. However, reduced expression of telomerases, *i.e.* the enzymes that maintain telomere length, has been shown to be a primary mechanism determining telomere shortening [17-

Table 1: Epigenetic effects of environmental contaminants.

POLLUTING AGENT	EFFECT	SETTING	REFERENCES
Particulate matter	Reduced telomere length in circulating blood leukocytes	Elderly smokers and traffic pollutants exposure	[14-16]
	Demethylation of *NOS2* gene and changes in the expression of miRNAs	Foundry workers long-term exposure to PM_{10}	[25-28]
Lead	LINE-1 hypomethylation	Cumulative exposure	[29, 30]
Arsenic	DNA methylation imbalance and hypermethylation of *p53* and *p16* promoters	Exposure to toxic level of arsenic in drinking water	[35-38]
Benzene	Hypermethylation in *p15* and hypomethylation of the *MAGEA1* cancer-antigen gene associated with increased risk of acute myelogenous leukemia	Gasoline station attendants and traffic police officers	[39, 40]
Polycyclic aromatic hydrocarbons	Hypermethylation of Alu, LINE-1 and *IL6*, hypomethylation of *p53* and *HIC1*, shortering of telomere length	Coke oven workers	[45, 47]
Persistent organic pollutants	Global DNA hypomethylation	Inuits from Greenland exposed to Environmental contaminants	[48]

19]. Interestingly, a recent study in a population of steel workers with high exposure to particulate matter did not find any evidence of changes in telomerase mRNA expression and promoter methylation in peripheral blood [20]. In the Normative Aging Study (NAS), a repeated measure investigation of elderly men in the Boston area, exposure to black carbon, a marker of traffic particles, was found to be associated with decreased blood DNA methylation in LINE-1 repetitive elements. More than 90% of all genomic 5-methylcytosines lie within CpG islands located in transposable repetitive elements, including the LINE-1 sequences, which are those most common and well-characterized. The presence of 5-methylcytosine limits the ability of retro-transposons to be activated and transcribed, and LINE-1 demethylation could result in increased retro-transposon activity and propagation of aberrant methylation to other genes [21]. As global blood DNA hypomethylation has been found in patients with cancer [22] and cardiovascular disease [23, 24], such changes may reproduce epigenetic processes related to disease development and represent mechanisms by which particulate air pollution affects human health [9]. Demethylation of the inducible Nitric Oxide Synthase (*NOS2*) has also been linked to particulate matter exposure. *NOS2* demethylation increases its expression and activity, which could in turn contribute to inflammation and oxidative stress generation. Tarantini *et al.* (2009) demonstrated that promoter methylation of the *NOS2* gene was lower in blood samples of foundry workers with well-characterized long-term exposure to particulate matter of 10 micrometers or less (PM_{10}). Also, PM_{10} was negatively associated with methylation in both Alu and LINE-1 sequences [25].

In the same study population, particulate matter exposure has been associated with changes in the expression of candidate miRNAs [26]. In this study, *miR-222* and *miR-21* expressions were increased after three days of exposure in the foundry, and such increases were correlated with the proportion of specific metal components in the particles. For example, *miR-222* expression was positively correlated with lead exposure [27, 28]. Moreover, *miR-21* expression was associated with blood levels of 8-hydroxyguanine, an oxidative stress marker, while *miR-146a* was negatively correlated with exposure to lead and cadmium. This report shows that air particles rich in lead and cadmium can disrupt miRNAs expression [26].

6.3. HEAVY METALS

6.3.1. Lead

Human exposure to lead can result in a wide range of biological effects depending upon the level and duration of exposure. Recently, Wright *et al.* (2010) found that LINE-1 DNA methylation was inversely associated with bone lead levels (a marker of long-term cumulative exposure) in a population of elderly men. Blood lead levels (a biomarker of recent exposure) were not associated with DNA methylation [29]. Pilsner *et al.* (2009) showed that prenatal lead exposure estimated from maternal bone levels was associated with alterations in DNA methylation of leukocytes obtained from umbilical cord samples. In particular, a negative correlation between exposure and genomic DNA methylation content in cord blood was observed. These results suggest that perinatal lead exposure might impact the epigenome of the developing fetus, thus causing gene reprogramming and potential disease susceptibility throughout the life course [30].

6.3.2. Arsenic

Arsenic is metabolized through repeated reduction and oxidative methylation. In the presence of high arsenic exposure, this detoxification process can compete for methyl donors with DNA methylation, thus causing perturbations in DNA methylation patterns [31]. An *in vitro* study on mammalian cells directly demonstrated that arsenic induced DNA hypomethylation, which was associated with chromosomal instability [32]. In addition, arsenite has been shown to increase the levels of both the repressive histone mark dimethylated H3K9 and the activating mark trimethylated H3K4, as well as to decrease the repressive mark trimethylated H3K27 in human lung carcinoma A549 cells [33].

In a study from India, significant DNA hypermethylation of *p53* and *p16* promoter regions was observed in blood DNA of subjects exposed to toxic levels of arsenic as compared to controls [34]. Gene promoter hypermethylation showed a dose-response relationship with arsenic measured in drinking water. Hypermethylation of *p16* was also noted in lung cancer samples of individuals with past exposure to chromate [35]. Unexpectedly, a recent study reported global dose-dependent hypermethylation of blood DNA in Bangladeshi adults with chronic arsenic exposure. This effect was modified by folate, suggesting that the arsenic-induced increases in DNA methylation were dependent on methyl availability [36]. However, the same group reported that lower blood DNA methylation was a risk factor for arsenic-induced skin lesions in a related Bangladeshi population [37].

Majumbar *et al.* (2010) monitored the variation of the capacity for methyl acceptance by DNA extracted from peripheral blood of individuals exposed to various doses of arsenic from drinking water in India and found a positive correlation between arsenic exposure and genomic hypermethylation. Taken together, these findings suggest that at least some of the effects of arsenic upon the epigenome can be detected in DNA of easily obtainable tissues such as blood [38].

6.4. ORGANIC COMPOUNDS

6.4.1. Benzene

Low-level benzene exposure induces methylation changes in peripheral blood DNA of gasoline station attendants and traffic police officers [39]. High-level exposure to benzene, on the other hand, has been associated with increased risk of acute myelogenous leukemia (AML) [40], which is characterized by aberrant global hypomethylation and gene-specific hypermethylation/hypomethylation. Moreover, exposure to airborne benzene was associated with a significant reduction in LINE-1 and Alu methylation. Airborne benzene was also associated with *p15* hypermethylation and hypomethylation of the *MAGEA1* cancer-antigen gene [39]. These findings show that low-level benzene exposure may induce altered DNA methylation, reproducing the aberrant epigenetic patterns found in malignant cells, which in most reports have been found to exhibit repetitive element hypomethylation as well as either hyper- or hypomethylation of specific genes, depending on the gene function. Also, benzene-associated demethylation of repetitive elements may help explain the epidemiological data linking benzene exposure with increased risk of multiple myeloma [41, 42], which also exhibits reduced methylation in Alu and LINE-1 repetitive elements [39]. Part of these results have been recently confirmed *in vitro* in human TK6 lymphoblastoid cells treated for 48h with hydroquinone, one of the active metabolites of benzene [43]. Hydroquinone induced global DNA hypomethylation at an intermediate level between melphalan (no effect) and etoposide (potent effect). These results suggest that hydroquinone may modify DNA methylation by mimicking the effects of alkylating agents and DNA topoisomerase II inhibitors [43].

6.4.2. Polycyclic Aromatic Hydrocarbons

Polycyclic aromatic hydrocarbons (PAHs) are chemicals that originate from the incomplete burning of organic substances including oil, coal, gas, garbage, tobacco or charbroiled meat. These compounds are usually found as a mixture of two or more chemicals. They are widely distributed and are considered lung carcinogens [44]. A study of blood DNA methylation in Polish coke oven workers exposed to polycyclic aromatic hydrocarbons found hypermethylation of Alu, LINE-1 and IL-6, and hypomethylation of *p53* and *HIC1* (hypermethylated in cancer 1) as compared with controls. DNA methylation changes were correlated with chromosomal instability and genetic damage such as micronuclei and anti-benzo[a]pyrene diolepoxide (anti-B[a]PDE)-DNA adduct levels. Overall, hypomethylation of the *p53* gene promoter had the highest correlation to PAH-exposure and showed the strongest association with micronuclei levels [45]. Interestingly, *p53* hypomethylation has been shown to predict lung cancer risk among male smokers [46]. In the same study population, Pavanello *et al.* (2010)

demonstrated that both chronic PAH exposure and *p53* hypomethylation were associated with shorter telomere length, an additional molecular characteristic that may contribute to malignant transformation [47].

6.4.3. Persistent Organic Pollutants

The relationship between plasma concentration of persistent organic pollutants (POPs) and blood DNA global methylation, estimated from Alu repeat elements was evaluated in 70 Greenlandic Inuit, a population presenting some of the highest reported levels of POPs worldwide. In this work, a significant inverse linear relationship with DNA methylation was found for DDT, DDE, β-BHC, oxychlordane, α-chlordane, mirex, several PCBs, and the sum of all POPs [48]. The levels found in this Arctic population, although extremely high, are comparable to those found in other regions. For example, an environmental assessment conducted in a Lacandon Maya community in the Southeast part of Mexico [49] showed levels of exposure to DDT comparable to those reported by Rusiecki *et al.* (2008).

6.5. A CONCEPTUAL MODEL FOR ENVIRONMENTAL EPIGENETICS

By definition, the environment includes all the physical, chemical and biological factors external to an individual. The concept of *"environmental epigenetics"* refers to the exposure to agents that impact the genome without affecting the nucleotide sequence but modify gene transcription through processes such as DNA methylation, histone modifications, and microRNA expression. Epigenetic mechanisms can provide cells and organisms with a form of molecular memory shaped by the environment. Epigenetic regulation can convert an environmental signal into a stable transcriptional response, which may then be perpetuated (inherited) even in the absence of the original stimulus [50]. However, the epigenetic effects of a single environmental agent may vary depending on concentration and time of exposure in addition to other factors such as individual genetic susceptibility, life stage, exposure to other pollutants or mixtures of pollutants and lifestyle. In Fig **1**, we propose a conceptual model for environmental epigenetics that we discuss in the following sections.

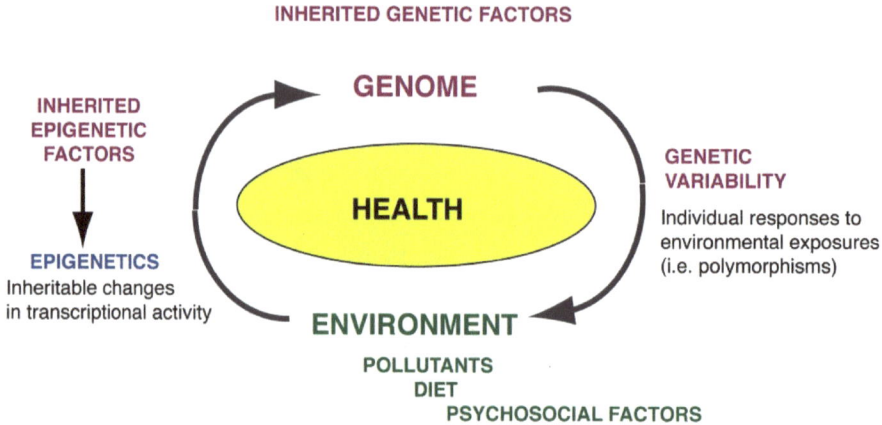

Figure 1: Interactions between epigenetics and the environment.

6.5.1. Genetic Variability

Some individuals have low risk of developing a disease as a result of an environmental exposure, while others are much more susceptible. For example, individuals that carry polymorphisms that make their cells less capable to respond to oxidative stress have been found in several investigations to be more susceptible to the cardiovascular and respiratory effects of air pollution, which produces health effects in humans, at least in part, through oxidative stress generation [51-53]. MiRNA expression has also been linked to redox balance control [54, 55] as well as to responses to cellular stress [56]. Recent evidence suggests that polymorphisms in genes that regulate miRNA processing could determine genetically regulated responses against environmental factors. For instance, Wilker *et al.* (2010) showed that the effects of air pollution on blood pressure were modified by single nucleotide polymorphisms (SNPs) in miRNA processing genes such as *DICER1*, *GEMIN4*, and DiGeorge critical region-8 (*DGCR8*) [57]. This example shows the tight inter-connections existing between genetic and epigenetic mechanisms.

6.5.2. Prenatal Exposure

Extensive evidence from animal studies and epidemiologic investigations shows that adult-onset diseases may have their origins *in utero*. Some of the effects of *in utero* exposures may persist across generations and may involve epigenetic mechanisms [58]. For instance, *in utero* exposure to tobacco smoking may produce epigenomic alterations that increase the risk for developing diseases in later life. *In utero* exposure to tobacco smoke has been shown to be associated with altered DNA methylation in the child buccal cells, including decreased LINE-1 methylation and hypermethylation of single CpG *loci* in eight genes detected through microarray hybridisation [59]. Toledo-Rodriguez *et al.* (2010) assessed DNA methylation of the brain-derived neurotrophic factor (*BDNF*) promoter -a gene that plays a role in brain development- in the blood of adolescents whose mothers smoked during pregnancy. The results showed *BDNF* hypermethylation, which was suggested to reflect potential epigenetic effects in the brain thus linking cigarette smoking to modifications in brain development and plasticity [60]. However, whether the smoking-induced *BDNF* hypermethylation in blood correlates with a similar alteration in the brain remains to be determined.

6.5.3. Exposure to Mixtures

Experimental studies investigate the effects of single chemicals and can identify with reasonable certainty specific epigenetic alterations associated with the exposure. In the real world, however, the same individual is usually exposed to several potential epigenetic toxicants. One major challenge for environmental epigenetics is to identify interactive effects among toxic agents [61]. Additive, synergistic, and antagonistic effects have not yet been sufficiently explored in epigenetics. Scenarios of multiple pollutant exposures abound in many settings. For instance, a recent exposure assessment campaign conducted in Mexico found high levels of both persistent organic pollutants and metals in nine populations of this country. It is noteworthy that in some of these communities the exposure level is comparable to those in reports that showed epigenetic disturbance [62].

6.5.4. Circadian Disruption

Stress response and circadian genes undergo epigenetic reprogramming by promoter methylation [63, 64]. The disruption of the circadian system may cause aberrant patterns of DNA methylation [65, 66]. Shiftwork is a common cause of circadian disruption [65, 66]. A recent study conducted in workers of two Italian chemical plants found no significant effect of nocturnal shiftwork upon DNA methylation imbalance of candidate genes [67]. However, blood samples from the individuals that had worked longer as shiftworkers showed Alu and IFN-γ promoter hypomethylation, a molecular change that may promote inflammation [68]. In subjects working the morning shift *TNF* hypomethylation was also observed, which can lead to a disregulation of the circadian system through increased expression of this cytokine [69]. However, the study did not collect multiple samples from each participant and was therefore limited in studying the chronobiological changes among shiftworkers. This example shows the need to consider the timing of DNA sampling in planning new epigenetic studies, as well as in analyzing existing data. In particular, some of the exposures, such as those occurring in occupational settings, might be associated with rotating shiftwork and disruption of the circadian rhythms.

FINAL CONSIDERATIONS

Epigenetic modifications are relatively stable over time and may be influenced by the environment. Exposure to pollutants may contribute to determine disease outcome *via* the epigenome. Experimental, clinical, and epidemiological studies of epigenetic phenomena have increased our understanding of the mechanisms of action by which environmental exposures modify gene expression. The contributions of *"environmental epigenetics"* to biomedicine might encompass the identification of the mechanisms through which the environment modulates gene expression, as well as the identification of new determinants of individual responses and susceptibility to environmental factors.

The ongoing development of newer approaches for experimental and human studies, and the increasing application of emergent technologies to the study of epigenetics promise to better our understanding of environmental diseases and find new means for their prevention.

REFERENCES

[1]   Baccarelli A, Bollati V. Epigenetics and environmental chemicals. Curr Opin Pediatr 2009; 21: 243-51.
[2]   Bollati V, Baccarelli A. Environmental epigenetics. Heredity 2010; 105: 105-12.

[3]   Anway MD, Leathers C, Skinner MK. Endocrine disruptor vinclozolin induced epigenetic transgenerational adult-onset disease. Endocrinology 2006; 147: 5515-23.

[4]   Dolinoy DC. The agouti mouse model. an epigenetic biosensor for nutritional and environmental alterations on the fetal epigenome. Nutr Rev 2008; 66(Suppl 1): S7-11.

[5]   Jirtle RL, Skinner MK. Environmental epigenomics and disease susceptibility. Nat Rev 2007; 8: 253–62.

[6]   Chuang KJ, Chan CC, Su TC, Lee CT, Tang CS. The effect of urban air pollution on inflammation, oxidative stress, coagulation, and autonomic dysfunction in young adults. Am J Respir Crit Care Med 2007; 176: 370-76.

[7]   Schwartz J. Air pollution and blood markers of cardiovascular risk. Environ Health Perspect 2001; 109(Suppl 3): 405-9.

[8]   Seaton A, MacNee W, Donaldson K, Godden D. Particulate air pollution and acute health effects. Lancet 1995; 345: 176-78.

[9]   Baccarelli A, Martinelli I, Zanobetti A, Grillo P, Hou LF, Bertazzi PA, *et al.* Exposure to particulate air pollution and risk of deep vein thrombosis. Arch Intern Med 2008; 168: 920-27.

[10]   Brook RD, Franklin B, Cascio W, Hong Y, Howard G, Lipsett M *et al.* Air pollution and cardiovascular disease. a statement for healthcare professionals from the Expert Panel on Population and Prevention Science of the American Heart Association. Circulation 2004; 109: 2655-71.

[11]   Peters A. Particulate matter and heart disease. Evidence from epidemiological studies. Toxicol Appl Pharmacol 2005; 207(2 Suppl): 477-82.

[12]   Samet JM, Dominici F, Curriero FC, Coursac I, Zeger SL. Fine particulate air pollution and mortality in 20 U.S. cities, 1987-1994. N Engl J Med 2000; 343: 1742-49.

[13]   Vineis P, Husgafvel-Pursiainen K. Air pollution and cancer. biomarker studies in human populations. Carcinogenesis 2005; 26: 1846-55.

[14]   Hoxha M, Dioni L, Bonzini M, Pesatori AC, Fustinoni S, Cavallo D, *et al.* Association between leukocyte telomere shortening and exposure to traffic pollution. a cross-sectional study on traffic officers and indoor office workers. Environ Health 2009; 8: 41.

[15]   McCracken J, Baccarelli A, Hoxha M, Dioni L, Coull B, Suh H, *et al.* Annual Ambient Black Carbon Associated with Shorter Telomeres in Elderly Men. Veterans Administration Normative Aging Study. Environ Health Perspect 2010; 118:1569.

[16]   Valdes AM, Andrew T, Gardner JP, Kimura M, Oelsner E, Cherkas LF, *et al.* Obesity, cigarette smoking, and telomere length in women. Lancet 2005; 366: 662-64.

[17]   Cong YS, Bacchetti S. Histone deacetylation is involved in the transcriptional repression of hTERT in normal human cells. J Biol Chem 2000; 275: 35665-68.

[18]   Li C, Wu MY, Liang YR, Wu XY. Correlation between expression of human telomerase subunits and telomerase activity in esophageal squamous cell carcinoma. World J Gastroenterol 2003; 9: 2395-99.

[19]   Yi X, Tesmer VM, Savre-Train I, Shay JW, Wright WE. Both transcriptional and posttranscriptional mechanisms regulate human telomerase template RNA levels. Mol Cell Biol 1999; 19: 3989-97.

[20]   Dioni L, Hoxha M, Nordio F, Bonzini M, Tarantini L, Albetti B *et al.* Effects of Short-Term Exposure to Inhalable Particulate Matter on Telomere Length, Telomerase Expression and Telomerase Methylation in Steel Workers. Environ Health Perspect 2010; 119:622-7.

[21] Asada K, Kotake Y, Asada R, Saunders D, Broyles RH, Towner RA *et al.* LINE-1 hypomethylation in a choline-deficiency-induced liver cancer in rats. dependence on feeding period. J Biomed Biotechnol 2006; 1: 17142-47.

[22] Ehrlich M. DNA methylation in cancer. too much, but also too little. Oncogene 2002; 21: 5400-13.

[23] Baccarelli A, Wright R, Bollati V, Litonjua A, Zanobetti A, Tarantini L *et al.* Ischemic heart disease and stroke in relation to blood DNA methylation. Epidemiology 2010; 21: 819-28.

[24] Castro, R., Rivera, I., Struys, E.A., Jansen, E.E., Ravasco, P., Camilo, M.E. *et al.* Increased homocysteine and S-adenosylhomocysteine concentrations and DNA hypomethylation in vascular disease. Clin. Chem 2003; 49: 1292–96.

[25] Tarantini L, Bonzini M, Apostoli P, Pegoraro V, Bollati V, Marinelli B *et al.* Effects of Particulate Matter on Genomic DNA Methylation Content and iNOS Promoter Methylation. Environ Health Perspect 2009; 117; 217-22.

[26] Bollati V, Marinelli B, Apostoli P, Bonzini M, Nordio F, Hoxha M *et al.* Exposure to metal-rich particulate matter modifies the expression of candidate microRNAs in peripheral blood leukocytes. Environ Health Perspect 2010; 118: 763-78.

[27] Sen CK, Gordillo GM, Khanna S, Roy S. Micromanaging vascular biology. tiny microRNAs play big band. J Vasc Res 2009; 46: 527–40.

[28] Suarez Y, Fernandez-Hernando C, Pober JS, Sessa WC. Dicer dependent microRNAs regulate gene expression and functions in human endothelial cells. Circ Res 2007; 100: 1164–73.

[29] Wright RO, Schwartz J, Wright RJ, Bollati V, Tarantini L, Park SK *et al.* Biomarkers of lead exposure and DNA methylation within retrotransposons. Environ Health Perspect 2010; 118: 790-95.

[30] Pilsner JR, Hu H, Ettinger A, Sánchez BN, Wright RO, Cantonwine D, *et al.* Influence of prenatal lead exposure on genomic methylation of cord blood DNA. Environ Health Perspect 2009; 117: 1466–71.

[31] Mass MJ, Wang L. Arsenic alters cytosine methylation patterns of the promoter of the tumor suppressor gene p53 in human lung cells. A model for a mechanism of carcinogenesis. Mutat Res 1997; 386: 263–77.

[32] Sciandrello G, Caradonna F, Mauro M, Barbata G. Arsenic-induced DNA hypomethylation affects chromosomal instability in mammalian cells. Carcinogenesis 2004; 25: 413-17.

[33] Zhou X, Sun H, Ellen TP, Chen H, Costa M. Arsenite alters global histone H3 methylation. Carcinogenesis 2008; 29: 1831-36.

[34] Chanda S, Dasgupta UB, Guhamazumder D, Gupta M, Chaudhuri U, Lahiri S, *et al.* DNA hypermethylation of promoter of gene p53 and p16 in arsenic exposed people with and without malignancy. Toxicol Sci 2006; 89: 431–37.

[35] Kondo K, Takahashi Y, Hirose Y, Nagao T, Tsuyuguchi M, Hashimoto M *et al.* The reduced expression and aberrant methylation of p16(INK4a) in chromate workers with lung cancer. Lung Cancer 2006; 53: 295-02.

[36] Pilsner JR, Liu X, Ahsan H, Ilievski V, Slavkovich V, Levy D *et al.* Genomic methylation of peripheral blood leukocyte DNA. influences of arsenic and folate in Bangladeshi adults. Am J Clin N 2007; 86: 1179-86.

[37] Pilsner JR, Liu X, Ahsan H, Ilievski V, Slavkovich V, Levy D *et al.* Folate deficiency, hyperhomocysteinemia, low urinary creatinine and hypomethylation of leukocyte DNA are risk factors for Arsenic-induced skin lesions. Environ Health Perspect 2009; 117: 254-60.

[38] Majumdar S, Chanda S, Ganguli B, Mazumder DN, Lahiri S, Dasgupta UB. Arsenic exposure induces genomic hypermethylation. Environ Toxicol 2010; 25: 315-18.

[39] Bollati V, Baccarelli A, Hou L, Bonzini M, Fustinoni S, Cavallo D *et al.* Changes in DNA methylation patterns in subjects exposed to low-dose benzene. Cancer Res 2007; 67: 876-80.

[40] Snyder R. Benzene and leukemia. Crit Rev Toxicol 2002; 32: 155-210.

[41] Costantini AS, Benvenuti A, Vineis P, Kriebel D, Tumino R, Ramazzotti V, *et al.* Risk of leukemia and multiple myeloma associated with exposure to benzene and other organic solvents. evidence from the Italian Multicenter Case-control study. Am J Ind Med 2008; 51: 803-11.

[42] Kirkeleit J, Riise T, Bratveit M, Moen BE. Increased risk of acute myelogenous leukemia and multiple myeloma in a historical cohort of upstream petroleum workers exposed to crude oil. Cancer Causes Control 2008; 19: 13-23.

[43] Ji Z, Zhang L, Peng V, Ren X, McHale CM, Smith MT: A comparison of the cytogenetic alterations and global DNA hypomethylation induced by the benzene metabolite, hydroquinone, with those induced by melphalan and etoposide. Leukemia 2010; 24: 986-91.

[44] Lewtas J. Air pollution combustion emissions. characterization of causative agents and mechanisms associated with cancer, reproductive, and cardiovascular effects. Mutat Res 2007; 636: 95-133.

[45] Pavanello S, Bollati V, Pesatori AC, Kapka L, Bolognesi C, Bertazzi PA, Baccarelli A. Global and gene-specific promoter methylation changes are related to anti-B[a]PDE-DNA adduct levels and influence micronuclei levels in polycyclic aromatic hydrocarbon-exposed individuals. Int J Cancer 2009; 125: 1692-97.

[46] Woodson K, Mason J, Choi SW, Hartman T, Tangrea J, Virtamo J *et al.* Hypomethylation of p53 in peripheral blood DNA is associated with the development of lung cancer. Cancer Epidemiol Biomarkers Prev 2001; 10: 69–74.

[47] Pavanello S, Pesatori AC, Dioni L, Hoxha M, Bollati V, Siwinska E *et al.* Shorter telomere length in peripheral blood lymphocytes of workers exposed to polycyclic aromatic hydrocarbons. Carcinogenesis 2010; 31: 216-21.

[48] Rusiecki JA, Baccarelli A, Bollati V, Tarantini L, Moore LE, Bonefeld-Jorgensen EC. Global DNA hypomethylation is associated with high serum-persistent organic pollutants in Greenlandic Inuit. Environ Health Perspect 2008; 116: 1547-52.

[49] Pérez-Maldonado IN, Athanasiadou M, Yáñez L, González-Amaro R, Bergman A, Díaz-Barriga F. DDE-induced apoptosis in children exposed to the DDT metabolite. Sci Total Environ 2006; 370: 343-51.

[50] Bourc'his D. Fundamentals of epigenetics. Bull Acad Natl Med 2010; 194: 271-81.

[51] Baccarelli A, Cassano PA, Litonjua A, Park SK, Suh H, Sparrow D, *et al.* Cardiac autonomic dysfunction. effects from particulate air pollution and protection by dietary methyl nutrients and metabolic polymorphisms. Circulation 2008; 117: 1802-09.

[52] Chahine T, Baccarelli A, Litonjua A, Wright RO, Suh H, Gold DR, *et al.* Particulate air pollution, oxidative stress genes, and heart rate variability in an elderly cohort. Environ Health Perspect 2007; 115: 1617-22.

[53] Park SK, O'Neill MS, Wright RO, Hu H, Vokonas PS, Sparrow D, *et al.* HFE genotype, particulate air pollution, and heart rate variability. a gene-environment interaction. Circulation 2006; 114: 2798-05.

[54] Brewer AC, Shah AM. Redox signalling and miRNA function in cardiomyocytes. J Mol Cell Cardiol 2009; 47: 2–4.

[55] Urbich C, Kuehbacher A, Dimmeler S. Role of microRNAs in vascular diseases, inflammation, and angiogenesis. Cardiovasc Res 2008; 79: 581–88.

[56] van Rooij E, Sutherland LB, Qi X, Richardson JA, Hill J, Olson EN. Control of stress-dependent cardiac growth and gene expression by a microRNA. Science 2007; 316: 575–79.

[57] Wilker EH, Baccarelli A, Suh H, Vokonas P, Wright RO, Schwartz J. Black carbon exposures, blood pressure, and interactions with single nucleotide polymorphisms in MicroRNA processing genes. Environ Health Perspect 2010; 118: 943-48.

[58] Woroniecki R, Gaikwad AB, Susztak K. Fetal environment, epigenetics, and pediatric renal disease. Pediatr Nephrol 2010; On line publication, ahead of press, 101007/s0046701017148.

[59] Breton CV, Byun HM, Wenten M, Pan F, Yang A, Gilliland FD. Prenatal tobacco smoke exposure affects global and gene-specific DNA methylation. Am J Respir Crit Care Med 2009; 180: 462-67.

[60] Toledo-Rodriguez M, Lotfipour S, Leonard G, Perron M, Richer L, Veillette S *et al.* Maternal smoking during pregnancy is associated with epigenetic modifications of the brain-derived neurotrophic factor-6 exon in adolescent offspring. Am J Med Genet B Neuropsychiatr Genet 2010; 153B. 1350-54 .

[61] Whittaker MH, Wang G, Chen XQ, Lipsky M, Smith D, Gwiazda R, Fowler BA. Exposure to Pb, Cd, and As mixtures potentiates the production of oxidative stress precursors. 30-day, 90-day, and 180-day drinking water studies in rats. Toxicol Appl Pharmacol 2010; On line publication, ahead of press, 101016/jtaap20101002.

[62] Trejo-Acevedo A, Díaz-Barriga F, Carrizales L, Domínguez G, Costilla R, Ize-Lema I *et al.* Exposure assessment of persistent organic pollutants and metals in Mexican children. Chemosphere 2009; 74: 974-80.

[63] Sahar S, Sassone-Corsi P. Circadian clock and breast cancer. a molecular link. Cell Cycle 2007; 6: 1329–31.

[64] Zhu Y, Zheng T, Stevens RG, Zhang Y, Boyle P. Does "clock" matter in prostate cancer?. Cancer Epidemiol Biomarkers Prev 2006; 15: 3–5.

[65] Haus E, Smolensky M. Biological clocks and shift work. circadian dysregulation and potential long-term effects. Cancer Causes Control 2006; 17: 489–500.

[66] Haus E. Circadian disruption in shiftwork is probably carcinogenic to humans. Chronobiol Int 2007; 24: 1255–56.

[67] Bollati V, Baccarelli A, Sartori S, Tarantini L, Motta V, Rota F, Costa G. Epigenetic effects of shiftwork on blood DNA methylation. Chronobiol Int 2010; 27: 1093-04.

[68] Cardoso FP, Viana MB, Sobrinho AP, Diniz MG, Brito JA, Gomes CC *et al.* Methylation pattern of the IFN-gamma gene in human dental pulp. J Endod 2010; 36: 642-46.

[69] Duguay D, Cermakian N. The crosstalk between physiology and circadian clock proteins. Chronobiol. Int 2009; 26: 1479–513.

www.ingramcontent.com/pod-product-compliance
Lightning Source LLC
Chambersburg PA
CBHW041705210326
41598CB00007B/533